Fractures of the Scapula

Robinson Esteves Pires • Pedro José Labronici
Vincenzo Giordano
Editors

Fractures of the Scapula

Current Management Concepts

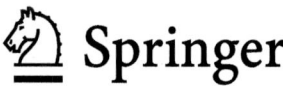

Editors
Robinson Esteves Pires
Department of the Locomotor Apparatus
Federal University of Minas Gerais
Belo Horizonte, Minas Gerais, Brazil

Pedro José Labronici
Department of General and
Specialized Surgery
Fluminense Federal University
Niterói, Brazil

Vincenzo Giordano
Orthopedics Department
Hospital Municipal Miguel Couto
Rio de Janeiro, Brazil

ISBN 978-3-031-58500-5   ISBN 978-3-031-58498-5   (eBook)
https://doi.org/10.1007/978-3-031-58498-5

© The Editor(s) (if applicable) and The Author(s), under exclusive license to Springer Nature Switzerland AG 2024

This work is subject to copyright. All rights are solely and exclusively licensed by the Publisher, whether the whole or part of the material is concerned, specifically the rights of translation, reprinting, reuse of illustrations, recitation, broadcasting, reproduction on microfilms or in any other physical way, and transmission or information storage and retrieval, electronic adaptation, computer software, or by similar or dissimilar methodology now known or hereafter developed.

The use of general descriptive names, registered names, trademarks, service marks, etc. in this publication does not imply, even in the absence of a specific statement, that such names are exempt from the relevant protective laws and regulations and therefore free for general use.

The publisher, the authors and the editors are safe to assume that the advice and information in this book are believed to be true and accurate at the date of publication. Neither the publisher nor the authors or the editors give a warranty, expressed or implied, with respect to the material contained herein or for any errors or omissions that may have been made. The publisher remains neutral with regard to jurisdictional claims in published maps and institutional affiliations.

This Springer imprint is published by the registered company Springer Nature Switzerland AG
The registered company address is: Gewerbestrasse 11, 6330 Cham, Switzerland

If disposing of this product, please recycle the paper.

Foreword

It is an honor to write a foreword for this important book on scapula fractures. The amount of information has exploded in the last two decades to improve diagnosis, management, approaches and outcomes of severe scapular fractures, and shoulder girdle injuries. As a resident, I saw only one formal Judet approach to the scapula with master surgeons, Steven Benirshke and Keith Mayo. These are relatively rare injuries and surgical indications were few at the time. As a young faculty, I approached my first severely comminuted, displaced scapula neck and body fracture with the formal Judet approach and thought that there must be a better way that is less invasive. This was in the early years of minimally invasive osteosynthesis and we described the modified Judet approach which I used for years, but others modified this modification to identify that the deltoid rarely needs to be released and that many fractures can be treated with even less invasive approaches. It also was noted that the reduction usually was to medialize the body and not to lateralize the glenoid. Further imaging studies confirmed that the glenoid remains in place as long as it is connected to the shoulder girdle and the scapula body lateralizes due to the pull of the posterior scapular muscles. This book reviews the increased knowledge of the last 20 years of scapula fracture diagnosis, approaches, and fixation strategies. We still have much to learn, but I believe these chapters increase our knowledge and understanding and guide us to improved outcomes for patients.

Nashville, TN, USA   William Obremskey

Foreword

In the craft of surgery the master word is simplicity
   —Berkeley George Andrew Moynihan (1865–1936)

It is an honor to introduce this well-written textbook. My good friends *Robinson E. Pires, Pedro J. Labronici, and Vincenzo Giordano*, superb Brazilian surgeons and educators, have worked closely with a first-class group of international contributors to deliver this book written in a comprehensive way dedicated to the ones involved with reconstruction of the scapula region. The publication is updated and reviews all the important aspects—from basic science to complex reconstruction—of this intricate and singular anatomic area.

Osteosynthesis was one of the greatest advances in orthopedic surgery—together with and arthroplasty and arthroscopy—of the twentieth century. The advances in this field take place every day around the globe and a textbook like this brings us the well-established principles and concepts.

From the nonoperative management to the still not well-recognized floating flail chest, the authors bring their own way of performing procedures to the benefit of the patients.

I congratulate the authors for this worthwhile addition to the trauma and shoulder surgery literature.

Passo Fundo, Brazil   Osvandre Lech
April 2024

Preface

The idea of this book stemmed from the collective expertise of three orthopaedic trauma surgeons deeply passionate about this subject. In recent decades, we have devoted a substantial portion of our professional careers to providing care for patients affected by this uncommon but challenging fracture.

Fractures of the Scapula: Current Management Concepts serves as a comprehensive guide for orthopaedic trauma surgeons, shoulder surgeons, thoracic surgeons, orthopaedic fellows and residents, medical students, physical therapists, and medical professionals involved in the care of patients with scapular fractures either isolated or associated with other injuries. This book aims to provide an in-depth exploration of the latest management strategies, surgical techniques, and rehabilitation protocols for these complex injuries.

In this book, renowned experts in the field from all over the globe share their insights and experiences, offering practical advice and evidence-based recommendations to navigate the diagnosis and treatment of scapular fractures effectively. Chapters cover a wide range of topics, including anatomy, embryology, classification systems, imaging, non-operative management, surgical indications, traditional and minimally invasive approaches, reduction and fixation strategies, rehabilitation protocols, and complications. The book will also delve into the concept of the floating shoulder and tackle a pertinent and emerging issue: periprosthetic scapular fractures subsequent to reverse shoulder arthroplasty.

As the understanding of scapular fractures continues to evolve, it is essential for healthcare providers to stay abreast of the latest advancements in the field. This book serves as a valuable resource, combining theoretical knowledge with practical guidance to enhance the care of patients with fractures of the scapula.

We hope that *Fractures of the Scapula: Current Management Concepts* will serve as a trusted companion for professionals involved with the care of patients sustaining scapular fractures, seeking to optimize their outcomes and improve their quality of life.

Belo Horizonte, Brazil	Robinson Esteves Pires
Niterói, Brazil	Pedro José Labronici
Rio de Janeiro, Brazil	Vincenzo Giordano

Acknowledgements

Acknowledgement by Vincenzo Giordano I dedicate this book first and foremost to my wife Érika and my daughters Carolina and Fernanda, whom I love deeply and who drive me every day to be a better person, professional, friend and, of course, husband and father. I also dedicate it to my parents José and Lúcia, brother Marcos, and aunt Sônia, who have always supported me in my professional decisions and helped me to remain firm in these choices. Finally, I dedicate it to my colleagues and friends at the Serviço de Ortopedia e Traumatologia Prof. Nova Monteiro–Hospital Municipal Miguel Couto, who have supported me for the last 30 years, and to the friends that orthopaedics has given me in life, including my two partners in this book, Robinson and Pedro, brothers in life.

Acknowledgement by Robinson Esteves Pires I would like to extend my appreciation to all the contributors who dedicated their time, expertise, and passion to make this book possible. Your invaluable insights and contributions have enriched the content and elevated the quality of this publication.

I am deeply thankful to the editorial team (Erica Ferraz, Anila Vijayan, and Jananee Ravichandran) for their dedication, professionalism, and tireless efforts throughout the entire process. Your attention to detail and commitment to excellence have been instrumental in shaping this book into its final form.

I am also grateful to my partners and special friends Vincenzo Giordano and Pedro Labronici for their commitment, engagement, assistance, expertise, and cooperation in all aspects of this project.

I would like to express my deepest gratitude to my mentors Prof. Márcio Ibrahim de Carvalho (*in Memoriam*), Prof. Fernando Baldy dos Reis, Prof. Marco Antônio Percope de Andrade, and Dr. Antônio Eleuterio Costa Pires, whose guidance, wisdom, and support have been instrumental in shaping my career and professional development.

I would also like to extend my thanks to the fellows, residents, and my partners in the orthopaedic surgery team at Felício Rocho Hospital, Orizonti Institute, and Risoleta Tolentino Neves Hospital, as well as to our patients, for making this dream possible.

Lastly, I want to express my heartfelt gratitude to my wife Ludmila and my daughters Laura and Gabriela for their unconditional support, patience, and encouragement during this long journey. I also would like to dedicate this book to my parents Helenice (*in Memoriam*) and Geraldo, as well as my brothers, Rodrigo and Robledo. Your unwavering support and guidance have been fundamental to my personal and professional development. I really hope that both patients and surgeons will benefit from the knowledge conveyed in this book.

Acknowledgement by Pedro José Labronici This is a very special moment for me, in which I express my deep gratitude, affection, and recognition to extraordinary individuals who played significant roles in my journey, especially for my two brothers at heart, Robinson Esteves and Vincenzo Giordano. Firstly, I dedicate this book to the surgeons passionate about the complexities of scapula fractures, a challenging and intricately treated injury.

Equally important, I dedicate this work to my beloved wife, Rosa, and my children, Ana Carolina, Gustavo, and Rodrigo. With their affection and unwavering support, they have been fundamental pillars that propelled me through this crucial phase of my life.

I also express my gratitude to my colleagues, whose constant support has been vital in my professional journey. To Hospital Santa Teresa (Congregação Santa Catarina) in Petrópolis, where I had the opportunity to enhance my professional knowledge, I extend my special acknowledgement.

Last but not least, I pay tribute "in memoriam" to my father, Aldo Labronici, who, besides being an orthopaedist, was my guide and mentor. I also dedicate this work to Donato D'angelo, who believed in my medical potential and imparted valuable lessons along the way. Their influences were crucial to my journey, and I am eternally grateful for their trust and guidance.

Contents

1	**Embryology, Anatomy, Biomechanics, Injury Mechanism, and Epidemiology of Scapular Fractures**................................ Robinson Esteves Pires, Pedro José Labronici, and Vincenzo Giordano	1
2	**Classification Systems for Scapular Fractures: How Useful Are They?**.. Robinson Esteves Pires, Pedro José Labronici, and Vincenzo Giordano	9
3	**Non-operative Management of Scapular Fractures: Patient Selection, Treatment Protocol, and Expected Outcomes**.... Robinson Esteves Pires, Pedro José Labronici, and Vincenzo Giordano	21
4	**Scapular Fractures in Children and Adolescents**................. Robinson Esteves Pires, Pedro José Labronici, and Vincenzo Giordano	27
5	**Approaches and Fixation Strategies for Scapular Fractures (Pitfalls and Opportunities): MIO Versus Conventional ORIF**..... Nathaniel E. Schaffer, Jaclyn M. Kapilow, and William T. Obremskey	33
6	**Special Considerations: Fractures of the Scapular Neck and Body**.. Kyle Auger, Jaclyn M. Jankowski, Richard S. Yoon, and Robinson Esteves Pires	45
7	**Special Considerations: Articular Involvement (Glenoid Fossa and Rim)**.................................. Vincenzo Giordano, David Rojas, and Robinson Esteves Pires	57

8	**Special Considerations: Fractures of the Coracoid Process and Acromion**	73
	Pedro José Labronici, Robinson Esteves Pires, and Vincenzo Giordano	
9	**Special Considerations: The Floating Shoulder—Myths and Reality**	89
	Fabio A. Suarez Romero and Federico Suarez Rodriguez	
10	**Special Considerations: The Floating Flail Chest—A New Entity**	101
	Robinson Esteves Pires, Vincenzo Giordano, and Pedro José Labronici	
11	**Special Considerations: Complex Scapular Fractures—Preoperative Planning and Fixation Strategies (Case Based)**	111
	Vincenzo Giordano, Robinson Esteves Pires, and Pedro José Labronici	
12	**Periprosthetic Scapular Fractures Following Reverse Shoulder Arthroplasty**	129
	Robinson Esteves Pires, Parag Shah, Chittaranjan Patel, and Vincenzo Giordano	
13	**Rehabilitation After Scapular Fractures**	137
	Andrea Lopes Sauers, Rita Ator, and Jaime González	
Index		145

About the Editors

Robinson Esteves Pires is a Professor of Orthopaedic Surgery and Traumatology at the Federal University of Minas Gerais, Belo Horizonte (MG), Brazil. Dr. Pires serves as the Chief of the Orthopaedic Trauma Service at Felício Rocho Hospital and Orizonti Institute. With a master's degree from the Federal University of São Paulo, Dr. Pires pursued his PhD and post-doctoral research at the Federal University of Minas Gerais. He completed a fellowship in Orthopaedic Trauma at the Federal University of São Paulo and served as visiting fellow at the University of Colorado (Denver Health Medical Center), University of California San Francisco (Orthopaedic Trauma Institute), and UC Davis (Sacramento, CA, USA). Dr. Pires is also an international AO Trauma Faculty and actively contributes to the Research Support Group of AO Trauma Latin America, while serving as a board member of AO Trauma Brazil. He is currently a member of the AO Trauma Lower Extremity Education Task Force.

Previously, he held the position of President of the Brazilian Society of Orthopedics and Traumatology (Minas Gerais State) and has been elected as President of the Brazilian Society of Orthopaedic Trauma for the year 2025. With a prolific academic career, Dr. Pires has authored several papers published in peer-reviewed journals and contributed to a substantial number of book chapters in the field of orthopaedic trauma.

Pedro José Labronici holds a master's degree in Medicine (Orthopedics and Traumatology) from the Federal University of Rio de Janeiro (UFRJ), a PhD in Orthopedics and Traumatology from the Federal University of São Paulo, Paulista School of Medicine (UNIFESP), and did his post-doctorate at the Fluminense Federal University (UFF). Dr. Labronici is currently Head of the Orthopedics and Traumatology Department at Santa Teresa Hospital. Dr. Labronici is an AO Trauma Faculty, a member of the Shoulder and Elbow Task Force of the AO International Trauma Group, and a board member of the Brazilian Orthopaedic Trauma Society. Dr. Labronici is a Full Professor at the Petrópolis School of Medicine. He is also an Associate Professor at the Universidade Federal Fluminense (UFF) and an Associate Professor at the Universidade Católica de Petrópolis. He also teaches in the postgraduate programme at the Universidade Federal Fluminense.

Vincenzo Giordano is an orthopaedic trauma surgeon and consultant at the Serviço de Ortopedia e Traumatologia Prof. Nova Monteiro—Miguel Couto Municipal Hospital since 1994. He has a master's degree and PhD from the Federal University of Rio de Janeiro and a post-doctorate from the Federal Fluminense University. He did a clinical fellow in orthopaedic trauma in 1999 at the University of Alabama at Birmingham and visiting fellows at the Klinik für Unfallchirurgie of the Medizinische Hochschule Hannover in 2002 and at the Klinik für Traumatologie of the Universitätsspital Zürich in 2005.

Dr. Giordano is currently the Research Officer for the AO Trauma Latin America and an International AO Trauma Faculty. He is fellow of the Brazilian College of Surgeons and responsible for the orthopaedic chapter. He is fellow of the Brazilian Academy of Military Medicine and responsible for the Surgical Clinics Section. He is past chair of the AO Trauma Brazil, the Brazilian Society of Orthopaedic Trauma, and the Brazilian Society of Orthopaedics and Traumatology (Rio de Janeiro State).

Dr. Giordano has several publications and book chapters in the area of orthopaedic trauma, many related to scapula fractures in partnership with the other authors of this book (R.E.S. and P.J.L.).

Chapter 1
Embryology, Anatomy, Biomechanics, Injury Mechanism, and Epidemiology of Scapular Fractures

Robinson Esteves Pires, Pedro José Labronici, and Vincenzo Giordano

1.1 Embryology of the Scapula

The development of the scapula is controlled by different genetic regulation in relation to the rest of the upper extremity. The embryology and genetic origin of the scapula are more similar to the spine, which explains the association between scapular and vertebral anomalies [1]. The knowledge of the embryology of the scapula is of paramount importance, since congenital anomalies, malformation, and abnormal scapular positioning may affect heart and respiratory functions and directly impair the function of the ipsilateral upper extremity [2].

Hita-Contreras et al. [3] reported three outgrowths of the mesenchymal condensation with irregular shape corresponding to the scapular body, the coracoid process, and a large mass of the acromion, scapular spine, and the humerus. However, the authors have not described whether the three outgrowths were connected. The morphogenesis of the coracoid process is different from the scapular body in several aspects. The coracoid ossification begins after the birth, differently from the scapular body. In average, between the 15th and 18th months after birth, ossification occurs in the middle of the coracoid process, which merges with the rest of the bone at 15 years of age [4–6].

R. E. Pires (✉)
Department of the Locomotor Apparatus, Federal University of Minas Gerais, Belo Horizonte, Minas Gerais, Brazil

P. J. Labronici
Department of General and Specialized Surgery, Fluminense Federal University, Niterói, Brazil

V. Giordano
Orthopedics Department, Hospital Municipal Miguel Couto, Rio de Janeiro, Brazil

© The Author(s), under exclusive license to Springer Nature Switzerland AG 2024
R. E. Pires et al. (eds.), *Fractures of the Scapula*,
https://doi.org/10.1007/978-3-031-58498-5_1

Müller and O'Rahilly [7] reported that the scapula is enlarged in the embryonic period, but it does not descend. Tanaka et al. [6] supported this finding in a morphometric study. Landmarks on the scapula and clavicle (superior angle, sternoclavicular joint, acromioclavicular joint, and glenoid fossa) remain in similar axial position, while only the axial position of the inferior angle decreases, which indicates that the scapula increases caudally, although it didn't descend.

1.2 Anatomy

The scapula is attached to the axial skeleton by the clavicle through the acromioclavicular and sternoclavicular joints, forming part of the shoulder girdle. The scapula rests on the posterior chest wall between the second and seventh costal ribs. The trapezius and the elevator scapulae are mainly responsible for holding the scapula in this position.

With an angle of approximately 30° between the scapula and the frontal plane, the scapula is primarily responsible for providing support to the humeral head.

The scapula presents a flat triangular shape divided into parts defined by the superior, medial, and lateral borders. In addition to the scapular spine and medial and lateral pillars, the scapula presents a three-dimensional anatomy which forms the scapular neck and the glenoid fossa. Posteriorly, the division between the scapular body and neck is marked by the spinoglenoid notch. The coracoid process is originated by the anterosuperior surface of the scapular neck. The glenoid fossa is concave and presents a pear-shaped articular surface with a prominent ring of fibrocartilage at its wider end (the glenoid labrum). The scapular spine divides the posterior surface of the scapula into the supra- and infraspinatus fossa. On the lateral aspect, the scapular spine becomes more elevated and ends on the acromion (Fig. 1.1). Knowing the distribution of the bony mass of the scapula is quite important, since implants are frequently applied on the surfaces which present a denser bone. The margins of the glenoid fossa, the scapular neck, and the base of the coracoid process are the regions with the highest bone density. Cancellous bone can be found only in the lateral angle of the scapula. The scapula presents two bony pillars, which cross from the glenoid to the scapular body, and transmit compression forces from the glenoid fossa.

The central zone of the scapula is a flat, extremely thin, and weak area. Most scapular body fractures cross this weak zone. Similarly, the central part of the scapular spine is also a relatively weak area, which justifies the fact of fracture lines generally reach this area [8]. The muscular complex that acts on the scapula should be divided into two main systems (scapuloaxial and scapulobrachial) [8]. The former connects the scapula with the axial skeleton, the spine, and the chest wall, being responsible for moving the scapula over the chest wall, whereas the latter is

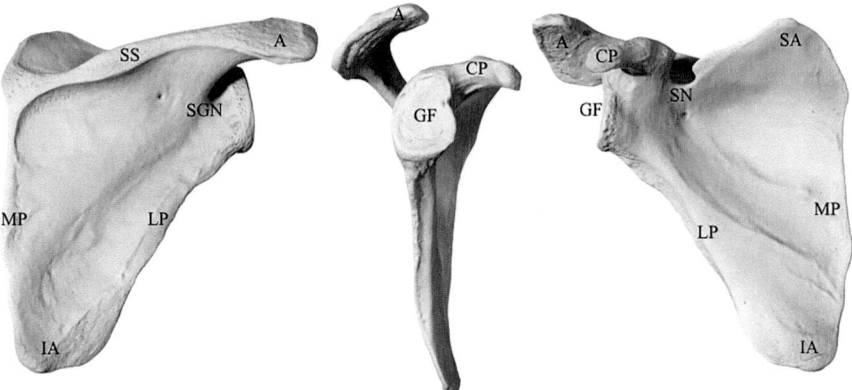

Fig. 1.1 Posterior, sagittal, and anterior views of the scapula. Acromion (A), coracoid process (CP), scapular spine (SS), later pillar (LP), medial pillar (MP), scapular notch (SN), spinoglenoid notch (SGN), inferior angle (IA), superior angle (SA), glenoid fossa (GN)

originated by the muscles arising from the scapula and attaching to the bones of the free part of the upper extremity, mainly the humerus, being responsible for controlling the movements of the glenohumeral joint [8].

In a total of 18 muscles attached to the scapula, only the subscapularis, supraspinatus, and infraspinatus originate from the broad surface of the scapula (Fig. 1.2). The rest of the muscles are attached to the borders of the scapula or its processes. Other muscles are responsible for reinforcing individual borders, angles, and processes by their attachments, such as the elevator scapulae at the superior angle, the rhomboid minor at the medial border at the level of the scapular spine posteriorly, and the rhomboid major and the latissimus dorsi at the inferior angle [8]. The teres minor originates from the upper half of the lateral border, and the teres major originates from the inferior angle and lateral border of the scapula. The serratus anterior muscle is attached to the medial border of the scapula, and the trapezius is attached to the scapular spine and the anterior rim of the acromion. The deltoid muscle arises from the posterior border of the acromion. The long head of biceps originates above the superior rim, while the long head of triceps originates from the inferior rim of the glenoid. The pectoralis minor originates from the central zone and the coracobrachialis from the tip of the coracoid process.

The suprascapular nerve crosses under the superior transverse scapular ligament and passes through the supraspinous fossa in association with the suprascapular artery and vein. Then, the neurovascular bundle penetrates the spinoglenoid notch, on the posterior surface of the scapular neck. The motor branches to the supraspinatus and infraspinatus muscles originate from the suprascapular nerve. An arterial anastomosis of the suprascapular artery and the scapular circumflex artery (Fig. 1.3) occurs on the lateral border of the scapula, around 2–3 cm distal to the glenoid fossa [8].

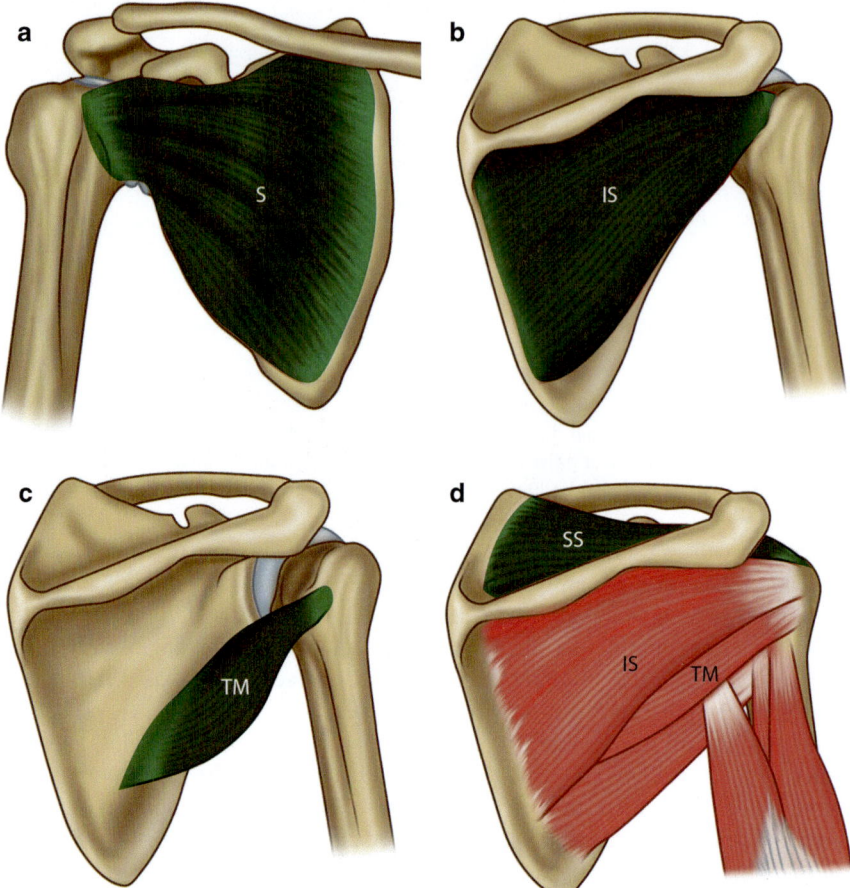

Fig. 1.2 Illustration of the muscles around the scapula. (**a**) Anterior view of the scapula. Subscapularis muscle (S). (**b**) Posterior view of the scapula. Infraspinatus muscle (IS). (**c**) Posterior view of the scapula. Teres minor muscle (TM). (**d**) Posterior view of the scapula. Supraspinatus muscle (SS), infraspinatus muscle (IS), teres minor muscle (TM)

Radiographic workup for scapular fractures may include the standard anteroposterior (AP) view, the true AP view (Grashey view), the axillary view, and the lateral view of the scapula (Y-view). Depending on the fracture location and associated injuries, other shoulder views should be included, such as the Stryker let view for coracoid process and anterior glenoid fossa rim, the AP and Zanca views for acromioclavicular joints, and the AP and 40° cephalad AP views for the clavicle (Fig. 1.4). Moreover, computed tomography (CT) scan has been shown to be useful to understand the morphology of the scapular fracture, to define the main fracture lines and secondary fracture lines, and to aid the surgical tactic when there is an indication for surgical management, as well as to demonstrate associated injuries.

Fig. 1.3 Illustration of the trajectory of the circumflex artery of the scapula (green) on the posterior aspect of the bone

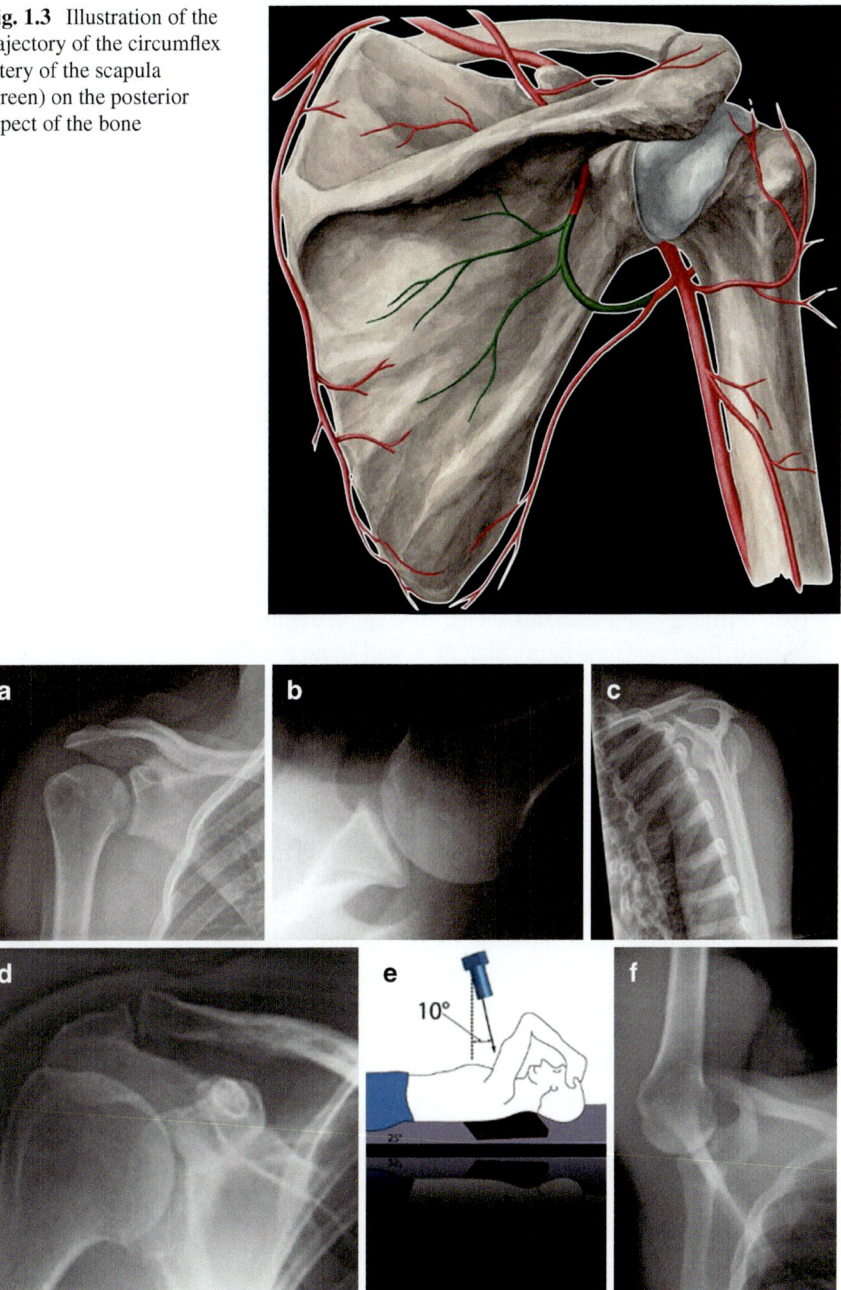

Fig. 1.4 Radiographic views of the shoulder. (**a**) True anteroposterior view (Grashey view) is obtained with the patient 35–45°, with the scapular body against the imaging detector. (**b**) Axillary view. (**c**) Lateral scapular (Y) view. (**d**) Zanca view for the acromioclavicular joint. (**e**) and (**f**) Illustration and radiograph using the Stryker let view for evaluation of coracoid process

1.3 Biomechanics, Injury Mechanism, and Epidemiology

The scapula is a relatively well protected bone due to its considerable mobility and location on the elastic chest wall [8]. Therefore, scapular fractures are rare, corresponding to 3% of all fractures [9–11]. Coimbra et al. [11] reported that patients presenting a scapular fracture are three times more likely to have a chest injury and twice as likely to have a spinal injury compared to other shoulder injuries after high-energy vehicular accidents. These authors also found that, comparing to other shoulder injuries in high-energy trauma, scapular fractures were more likely to occur in a rollover mechanism or side car impact, while other shoulder injuries were more likely to occur due to frontal impact. Moreover, scapula fractures were caused by the vehicular occupant hitting the interior side (vehicle pillars, door panel, or door hardware/armrest) of the vehicle, whereas the occupants with other shoulder injuries were more likely to be injured by other vehicle components in frontal crashes.

Didactically, from the epidemiological point of view, scapular fractures may be divided into four major groups:

1. First group: Polytrauma patients suffering high-energy injuries usually due to road traffic accidents. In this scenario, scapula fractures are generally associated to head, thoracic (ribs, lung), abdomen, and spine injuries. The spectrum of scapular injury can range from a complex fracture pattern to a relatively simple one, incidentally diagnosed in the imaging workup of chest trauma.
2. Second group: The second group corresponds to patients with medium-energy trauma usually caused by a bicycle fall or a slowly travelling motorcycle or similar. The scapula and the shoulder girdle injuries usually dominate the clinical scenario, and associated injuries may also be present.
3. Third group: This group depicts open fractures of the scapula caused by gunshot injuries (Fig. 1.5). The military population has up to 20 times higher risk of open scapula fractures, and most of these fractures are comminuted and present associated injuries [12]. In cases of open scapular fractures caused by cold weapon, the fracture is most often located on the scapular body, scapular spine, or processes (more likely the acromion).
4. Fourth group: This group corresponds to geriatric fractures due to low-energy trauma with direct impact on the shoulder or pathological scapular fractures (e.g., bone metastasis, osteodystrophy) [8–13]. Another growing fracture pattern is the periprosthetic fracture of the scapular spine or acromion in patients following reverse shoulder arthroplasty (RTSA) [8, 13–15]. The incidence of scapular fractures occurring after RTSA has been reported to be between 5.8% and 10.2% [14, 15].

Scapular fractures can be caused by transmitted forces, with the humeral head acting as a hammer. Arm position determines the fracture pattern and the degree of displacement. In abduction and external rotation, the humeral head is driven against the inferior glenoid, which is fractured usually together with a part of the lateral

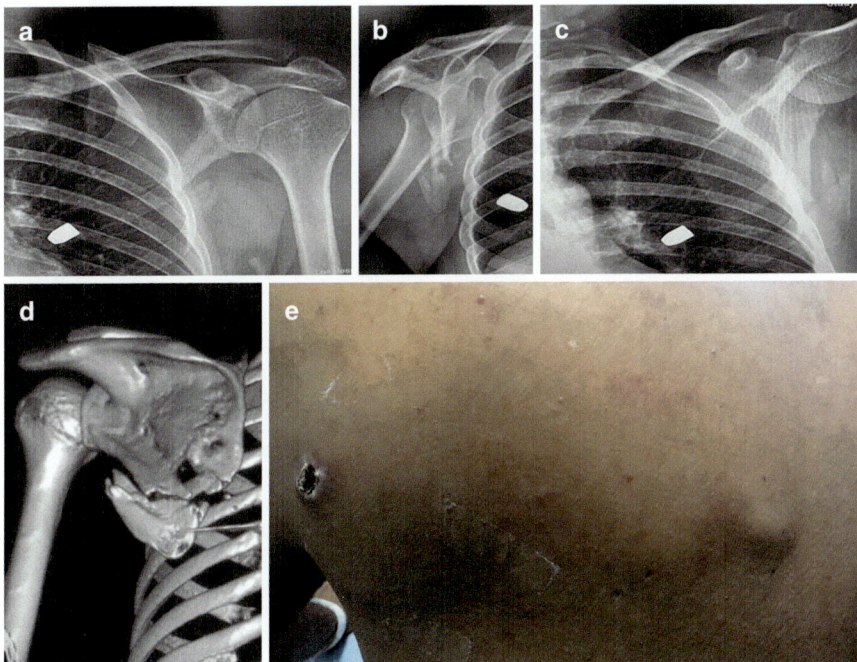

Fig. 1.5 Figure 1.5 depicts a case of a 30-year-old patient who suffered a low-energy gunshot injury on the posterior aspect of the left shoulder. Observe the radiographs in anteroposterior (**a**), lateral (**b**), and axillary (**c**) views showing the inferior angle fracture and the projectile. CT scan with 3D reconstruction showing the fracture of the inferior angle of the scapula caused by the gunshot injury (**d**). Clinical aspect of the posterior surface of the left shoulder (**e**). Observe the subcutaneous pathway of the gunshot

pillar of the scapula. In adduction, a force directed on the elbow along the axis of the humeral shaft proximally dislocates the humeral head proximally, which hits the coracoid process or the acromion. Posterior or anterior dislocation of the shoulder may result in a fracture of the respective rim of the glenoid, caused by the impact of the humeral head associated with internal or external rotation, respectively. More rarely, scapular fractures may result of an endogenous cause of violent muscle contracture (e.g., epileptic seizure or electrical injury), which generally produces posterior dislocation of the fragments [8]. Another rare and distinct fracture pattern is the fracture of the inferior angle of the scapula. Alder-Price et al. [16] reported a bimodal distribution of this injury with high-energy trauma accounting for younger males, and low-energy trauma in the elderly population. Males were found to be affected more commonly than females in a 5:2 ratio. The anterior displacement or angulation seen in fractures of the inferior angle of the scapula occurs because of the muscles force attached to the inferior angle of the scapula. The inferior angle thoracic surface is attached to serratus anterior medially and laterally. The posterior surface is attached to rhomboid major medially and teres major laterally. Additionally, the inferior tip is attached to latissimus dorsi in 43% of the population.

Yimam et al. [17] performed a three-dimensional computerized fracture mapping and observed that scapular fractures propagated through multiple zones. The three most common exit zones were the lateral (69%), medial (67%), and superior borders (60%). The superior lateral border, medial base of the scapula spine, spinoglenoid notch, and mid-superior border were the most frequent zones of fracture in the scapular body. Simple-pattern intra-articular fractures (transverse or oblique) were the most common (92%) fracture types in the glenoid region.

References

1. Williams MS. Developmental anomalies of the scapula-the "omo"st forgotten bone. Am J Med Genet A. 2003;120:583–7.
2. Monfort K, Case-Smith J. The effects of a neonatal positioner on scapular rotation. Am J Occup Ther. 1997;51:378–84.
3. Hita-Contreras F, Sánchez-Montesinos I, Martínez-Amat A, Cruz-Diaz D, Barranco RJ, Roda O. Development of the human shoulder joint during the embryonic and early fetal stages: anatomical considerations for clinical practice. J Anat. 2018;232:422–30.
4. O'Rahilly R, Gardner E. The initial appearance of ossification in staged human embryos. Am J Anat. 1972;134:291–301.
5. Schaefer M, Black S, Scheuer L. Juvenile osteology: a laboratory and field manual. 1st ed. Burlington: Elsevier Inc; 2009.
6. Tanaka S, Sakamoto R, Kanahashi T, Yamada S, Imai H, Yoneyama A, et al. Shoulder girdle formation and positioning during embryonic and early fetal human development. PLoS One. 2020;15(9):e0238225.
7. Müller F, O'Rahilly R. Somitic-vertebral correlation and vertebral levels in the human embryo. Am J Anat. 1986;177:3–19.
8. Bartoníček J, Tuček M, Naňka O. Scapular fractures. In: Textbook of shoulder surgery. 1st ed. Cham: Springer Nature; 2019. p. 55–73.
9. Baldwin KD, Ohman-Strickland P, Mehta S, Hume E. Scapula fractures: a marker for concomitant injury? A retrospective review of data in the national trauma database. J Trauma. 2008;65:430–5.
10. Veysi VT, Mittal R, Agarwal S, et al. Multiple trauma and scapula fractures: so what? J Trauma. 2003;55:1145–7.
11. Coimbra R, Carol Conroy C, Tominaga GT, Bansal V, Schwartz A. Causes of scapula fractures differ from other shoulder injuries in occupants seriously injured during motor vehicle crashes. Injury. 2020;4:151–5.
12. Tüzün HY, Erşen O, Arsenishvili A, Türkkan S, Kürklü M. Functional outcomes of internal fixation of scapula fractures due to high-velocity gunshot injuries. Eur J Trauma Emerg Surg. 2022;48(3):1987–92.
13. Cole PA Jr, Jacobson AR, Cole PA. Open reduction and internal fixation of scapula fractures in a geriatric series. Geriatr Orthop Surg. 2015;6(3):180–5.
14. Crosby LA, Hamilton A, Twiss T. Scapula fractures after reverse total shoulder arthroplasty: classification and treatment. Clin Orthop Relat Res. 2011;469:2544–9.
15. Stevens CG, Murphy MR, Stevens TD, Bryant TL, Wright TW. Bilateral scapular fractures after reverse shoulder arthroplasties. J Shoulder Elb Surg. 2015;24:e50–5.
16. Alder-Price AC, Pilch W, Zhuang CB, McLean J, Bain GI. Inferior angle of scapula fractures: a retrospective case series. J Orthop Surg. 2022;30(1):1–5.
17. Yimam HM, Dey R, Rachuene PA, Kauta NJ, Roche SJL, Sivarasu S. Identification of recurring scapular fracture patterns using 3-dimensional computerized fracture mapping. J Shoulder Elb Surg. 2022;31:571–9.

Chapter 2
Classification Systems for Scapular Fractures: How Useful Are They?

Robinson Esteves Pires, Pedro José Labronici, and Vincenzo Giordano

2.1 Introduction

There are several classification systems for scapular fractures based on different anatomical aspects. Basically, scapular fractures can be divided into extra- and intra-articular fracture patterns. Extra-articular fractures of the coracoid process, acromion process, neck, body, and spine account for most scapular fractures, while intra-articular fractures constitute 10–30% of all scapular fractures.

Among extra-articular fractures, scapular body fractures are the most common fracture site, accounting for 35–45% of scapula fractures, followed by scapular neck fractures, accounting for 26–29% of scapula fractures. Furthermore, fractures of the coracoid process account for 2–13% of scapula fractures, while acromion fractures account for 8–16% of scapula fractures.

R. E. Pires (✉)
Department of the Locomotor Apparatus, Federal University of Minas Gerais, Belo Horizonte, Minas Gerais, Brazil

P. J. Labronici
Department of General and Specialized Surgery, Fluminense Federal University, Niterói, Brazil

V. Giordano
Orthopedics Department, Hospital Municipal Miguel Couto, Rio de Janeiro, Brazil

© The Author(s), under exclusive license to Springer Nature Switzerland AG 2024
R. E. Pires et al. (eds.), *Fractures of the Scapula*,
https://doi.org/10.1007/978-3-031-58498-5_2

2.2 Classification Systems for Scapula Fractures

2.2.1 Jean Louis Petit Classification

To the best of our knowledge, this was the first classification system described for scapular fractures. The Petit classification [1] divides the scapula into three regions: body, neck, and processes (coracoid and acromion). Petit further subdivided the scapular body fracture into longitudinal, transverse, and oblique.

2.2.2 AO/OTA Classification

The AO/OTA classification system for scapular fractures was revisited in 2018. In this classification system, scapula is codified as 14. The AO/OTA divides scapula fractures in three main groups: scapula process fractures (type A), scapula body fractures (type B), and fractures involving the glenoid fossa (type F). Each superordinate category consists of various subtypes, e.g., glenoid fractures are divided into 11 possible fracture patterns. Qualifiers should be included according to the fracture location [2] (Fig. 2.1).

2.2.3 Euler and Rüedi Classification

Another relatively popular scapular fracture classification is the Euler and Rüedi classification [3]. In the subdivision for glenoid fractures, Euler and Rüedi distinguished six different types of fracture patterns. Moreover, types of fracture patterns can be combined (Fig. 2.2). Huflage et al. [3] evaluated the reproducibility of the AO/OTA and Euler Rüedi classifications. They observed that the AO/OTA classification is most suitable to categorize intra-articular scapula fractures with glenoid involvement, whereas the classification system of Euler and Rüedi appears to be superior in extra-articular injury patterns with fractures involving only the scapula body, spine, coracoid process, and acromion.

2.2.4 Harvey Classification

This classification system was developed based on two codes, one to describe fractures involving the fossa or body, and the other to independently describe process fractures. It was created with more in-depth subcategories for fracture classification. The articular segment area involves the glenoid fossa and the articular rim and is limited superiorly by a line joining the superior articular rim to the lateral border of

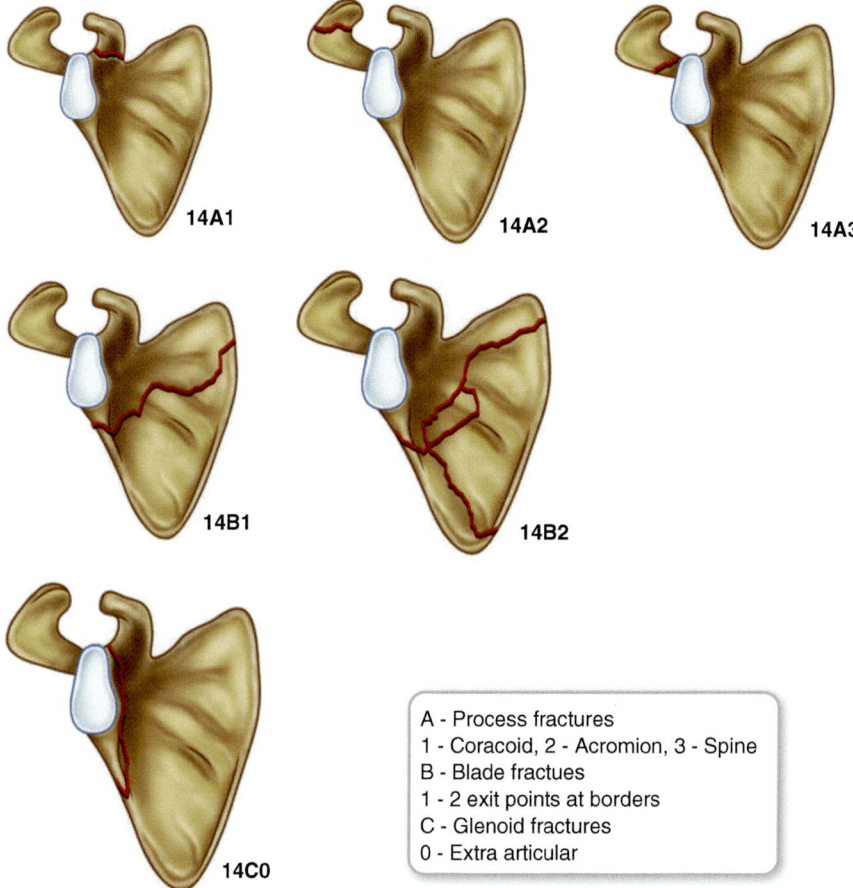

Fig. 2.1 AO/OTA classification system for scapular fractures

the suprascapular notch and from that point medially by a line parallel to the plane of the glenoid fossa. The process fractures include the acromion and the coracoid. The acromion is lateral to the plane of the glenoid fossa, and the coracoid is defined by the superior limit of the articular segment. The body is defined as the area that is neither process nor articular segment. The articular fractures (F) are divided into the following subtypes: F0—fracture of the articular segment, not through the glenoid fossa (the fossa is not attached to any part of the scapula body); F1—simple pattern: rim, transverse, and oblique fractures (fracture involves the glenoid fossa); and F2— multifragmentary joint fracture (fracture involves the glenoid fossa with three or more articular fragments). Body fractures (B) can involve the lateral, medial, and superior borders separately and are described with 1 or more fracture lines running through the body. Scapular body fractures are subdivided into B1—simple fracture patterns with fracture lines that exit at 2 or less points; and B2—complex fracture

A	B	C	D	E
Scapula body fractures	Scapula process fractures	Scapula neck fractures	Articular fractures	Combined fractures
Isolated or multifragmentary	B1 Spine fracture B2 Coracoid fracture B3 Acromion fracture	C1 Anatomical neck fracture C2 Surgical neck fracture C3 Surgical neck fracture with a) Clavicle fracture b) Ligament tear	D1 Glenoid rim fracture D2 Glenoid fossa with a) Inferior glenoid fragment b) Horizontal split fracture c) Coracoglenoid block formation d) Communicated fractures D3 Scapula neck and body	Concomitant humeral head fractures

Fig. 2.2 Euler and Rüedi classification system

patterns with fracture lines exiting at 3 or more points. In fracture patterns involving the articular segment, one of the exits is considered in the articular segment [4] (Fig. 2.3).

2.2.5 Ada and Miller Classification

Ada and Miller [5] developed a classification system based on a retrospective review of 116 scapular fractures. The authors named fractures of the acromion and coracoid process in types I and II, respectively. Three types of neck fractures were also described, according to the course of fracture lines: Type IIA (fractures of the surgical neck); type IIB (transpinous scapular neck fractures); and type IIC (transverse fractures of the scapular body) [6] (Fig. 2.4).

2.2.6 Goss Classification

Goss [7] modified the Ada and Miller [5] classification system, excluding transpinous scapular neck fractures, and including fractures of the anatomical neck. The author named the fracture of neck inferior to scapula spine as type IIC [6] (Fig. 2.5).

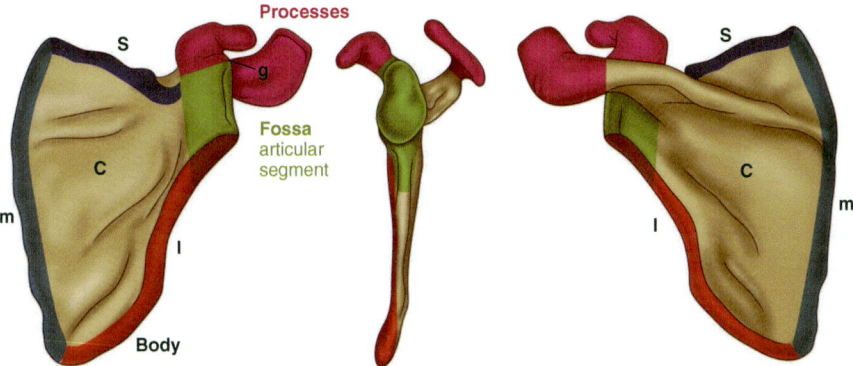

Fig. 2.3 Harvey et al. classification system for scapular fractures

Fig. 2.4 Ada and Miller classification system

Type I	Acromion, scapular spine, coracoid process fractures
Type II	Scapular neck fractures
Type III	Glenoid fractures
Type IV	Scapular body fractures

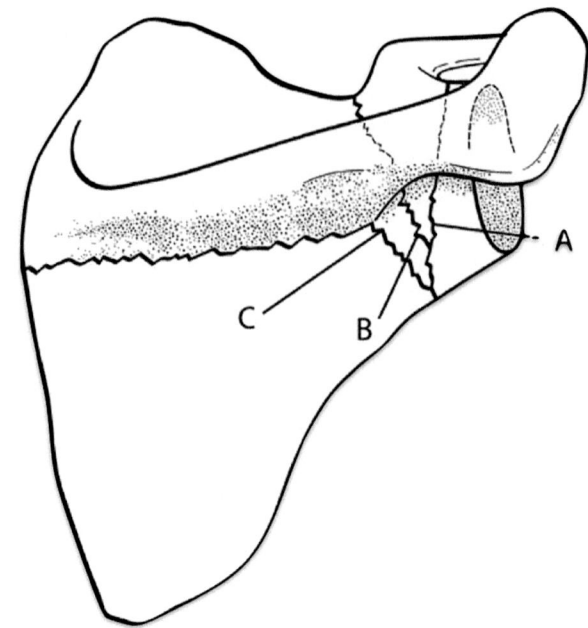

Fig. 2.5 Goss classification system. (**a**) Fracture of the anatomical neck. (**b**) Fracture of the surgical neck. (**c**) Fracture of the neck, inferior to the scapular spine

2.2.7 Hardegger Classification

Hardegger et al. [8] classification system is quite similar to the Ada and Miller system and defines two types of neck and two types of glenoid fractures.

2.2.8 Bartoníček Classification for Scapular Body Fractures

Bartoníček et al. [9] described a classification system for fractures of scapula body based on the findings of the CT scans of 187 patients. These authors divided the scapular body fractures into three major groups: fractures of the spinal pillar; fractures of the lateral pillar (2-part, 3-part, and comminuted fractures); and fractures of both pillars (fractures involving the medial third of the spinal pillar and fractures involving the central part of the spinal pillar) [6, 9, 10].

2.2.9 Ideberg Classification

The Ideberg et al. [11] classification is the most used system for glenoid cavity fractures of the scapula. The authors grouped glenoid fractures based on a case series of 338 patients. This classification received later modifications by Goss et al. [12] and Mayo et al. [13] and divides the fracture patterns into glenoid rim fractures (type I) and glenoid fossa fracture with increasing degrees of scapular neck and body involvement (types II–VI). Type I fractures are vertically oriented fractures of the anterior or posterior glenoid rim and are larger than a typical bony Bankart lesion. They occur with a laterally directed impact of the humeral head on the glenoid rim, rather than anterior or posterior humeral head translation. Type II–IV fractures are described by a transverse intra-articular fracture that exits through the lateral, superior, and medial scapular border, respectively. Type V fractures are combinations of types II–IV. Types III and V fractures are the most likely to be accompanied by a second injury in the superior shoulder suspensory complex, resulting in a highly unstable shoulder (floating shoulder). Type VI fractures are severely comminuted at the articular surface [12] (Fig. 2.6).

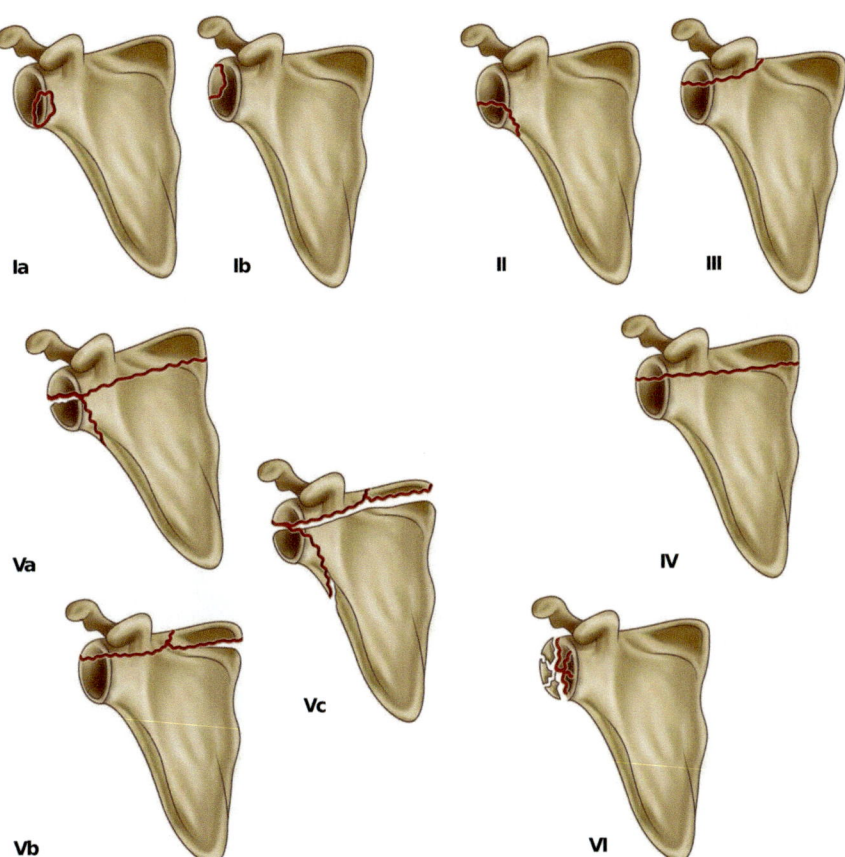

Fig. 2.6 Illustration of the Ideberg classification system. Type I fractures involve the anterior (Ia) or posterior (Ib) glenoid rim. Type II–IV fractures are transverse through the glenoid and exit through the lateral (II), superior (III), or medial (IV) scapula. Type V fractures are combinations of types II–IV, including lateromedial (Va), superomedial (Vb), and superomediolateral (Vc) scapular extension. Type VI fractures are highly comminuted at the articular surface and are usually irreparable

2.2.10 Ogawa Classification System for Coracoid Process Fractures

Several classification systems were proposed for coracoid process fractures. In the Ogawa [14] classification system, the type I fracture is proximal to the coracoclavicular ligament attachment, while the type II fracture is distal (Fig. 2.7).

2.2.11 Eyres Classification System

Eyres et al. [15] proposed a more detailed classification system based on a review of 12 coracoid process fractures. In this classification, coracoid fractures are divided into five types and subgrouped into A or B, according to the presence or absence of associated injuries to the clavicle or its ligamentous connection that affects scapular stability, respectively. Type I coracoid fracture involves the tip or epiphyseal area; type II is a midprocess fracture; type III is a fracture of the basis of the coracoid process; type IV is a fracture of the superior body of the scapula; and type V is a fracture extending into the glenoid fossa (Fig. 2.8).

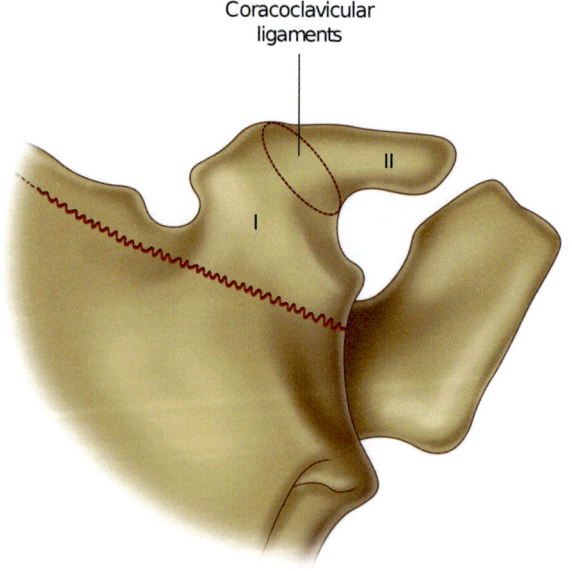

Fig. 2.7 Illustration of the Ogawa classification system. Type I fracture is proximal to the coracoclavicular ligament attachment, while the type II fracture is distal

Fig. 2.8 Illustration depicting the Eyres classification system for coracoid process fractures. Type I is a tip or epiphyseal fracture, type II is a midprocess fracture, type III is a basal fracture, type IV is a fracture with involvement of the superior scapular body, and type V is a fracture with extension in the glenoid fossa

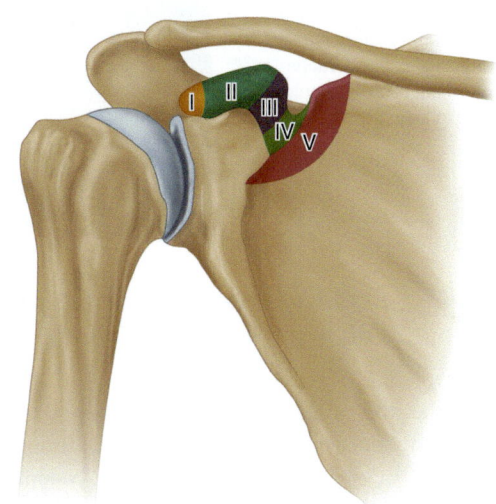

2.2.12 Bartoníček Classification System for Coracoid Process Fractures

Bartoníček et al. [16] developed a classification based on 3D-CT reconstructions. Type I is a fracture of apex; type II is a fracture of beak; type III is a fracture of base; and type IV is a comminuted fracture pattern of the coracoid process.

2.2.13 Kuhn Classification System for Acromion Fractures

Kuhn et al. [17], in a case series of 27 acromion fractures managed non-operatively, classified acromion fractures into three types. Type I is a minimally displaced acromion fracture; type II is a laterally displaced fracture with no constraint in the subacromial space; and type III is a displaced fracture of the acromion with reduction of the subacromial space. Type I acromion fractures are subdivided into type IA (avulsion fracture) and type IB (true acromion fracture).

2.2.14 Ogawa and Naniwa Classification System for Acromion Fractures

Ogawa and Naniwa [18] proposed a simple and anatomical classification. Type I represents a fracture in the lateral region of the acromion; and type II represents a fracture medial to the acromion with a descending line toward the spinoglenoid notch.

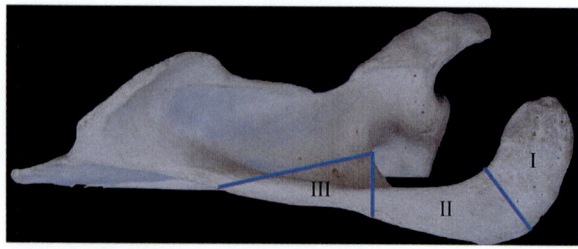

Fig. 2.9 Illustration of the Levy classification system for periprosthetic fractures following reverse shoulder arthroplasty

2.2.15 Levy Classification for Periprosthetic Fractures Following Reverse Shoulder Arthroplasty

With the dizzying growth in the number of reverse shoulder arthroplasties (RSA), periprosthetic scapular spine or acromial fracture is a rare but emerging complication. The Levy et al. [19] classification system is based on the origin of the deltoid (Fig. 2.9). The anterior and middle portions of the deltoid are involved in Levy type 1 fractures, the middle and part of the posterior deltoid are involved in Levy type 2 fractures, and Levy type 3 fractures involve the middle and entire posterior deltoid origin. In Levy type 1 fracture, scapulothoracic motion is normal and preserved, whereas RSA biomechanics may be affected when a larger portion of the deltoid insertion is disrupted.

This anatomic classification is universally used to guide the treatment.

2.3 Conclusion

Even knowing that there is no ideal classification system for scapula fractures, our preferred systems are Bartoníček et al. [9] for scapular body fractures, Ideberg et al. [11] for glenoid fossa and rim fractures, Bartoníček et al. [16] for coracoid process fractures, Kuhn et al. [17] for acromion fractures, and Levy et al. [19] for periprosthetic scapular fractures following reverse shoulder arthroplasty.

References

1. Petit JL. Traité des Maladies des Os, tome second. Paris: Charles Etienne Hochereau; 1723. p. 122–38.
2. Meinberg EG, Agel J, Roberts CS, Karam MD, Kellam JF. Fracture and dislocation classification compendium-2018. J Orthop Trauma. 2018;32:S1–S170.
3. Huflage H, Fieber T, Christian Farber C, Knarr J, Veldhoen S, Jordan MC, Gilbert F, Bley TA, Meffert RH, Jan-Peter Grunz JP, Schmalzl J. Interobserver reliability of scapula fracture classifications in intra- and extra-articular injury patterns. BMC Musculoskelet Disord. 2022;23:189.

4. Harvey E, Audigé L, Herscovici DH Jr, Agel J, Madsen JE, Babst R, Nork S, Kellam J. Development and validation of the new international classification for scapula fractures. J Orthop Trauma. 2012;26(6):364–9.
5. Ada JR, Miller ME. Scapular fractures. Analysis of 113 cases. Clin Orthop Relat Res. 1991;269:174–80.
6. Pires RE, Giordano V, Mendes de Souza FS, Labronici PJ. Current challenges and controversies in the management of scapular fractures: a review. Patient Saf Surg. 2021;15(6):1–18.
7. Goss TP. Fractures of glenoid neck. J Shoulder Elb Surg. 1994;3:42–52.
8. Hardegger F, Simpson LA, Weber BG. The operative treatment of scapula fractures. J Bone Joint Surg. 1984;66-B:725–31.
9. Bartonicek J, Klika D, Tucek M. Classification of scapular body fractures. Rozhl Chir. 2018;97(2):67–76.
10. Bartoníček J, Tuček M. Infraglenoid fracture of the scapular neck fact or myth? Rozhl Chir. 2019;98(7):273–6.
11. Ideberg R, Grevsten S, Larsson S. Epidemiology of scapular fractures incidence and classification of 338 fractures. Acta Orthop Scand. 1995;66:395–7.
12. Goss TP. Fractures of the glenoid cavity. J Bone Joint Surg Am. 1992;74(2):299–305.
13. Mayo KA, Benirschke SK, Mast JW. Displaced fractures of the glenoid fossa. Results of open reduction and internal fixation. Clin Orthop Relat Res. 1998;347:122–30.
14. Ogawa K, Yoshida A, Takahashi M, et al. Fractures of the coracoid process. J Bone Joint Surg Br. 1997;79:17–9.
15. Eyres KS, Brooks A, Stanley D. Fractures of the coracoid process. J Bone Joint Surg Br. 1995;77:425–8.
16. Bartoníček J, Tuček M, Strnad T, et al. Fractures of the coracoid process—pathoanatomy and classification: based on thirty nine cases with three dimensional computerised tomography reconstructions. Int Orthop. 2021;45(9):1009–15.
17. Kuhn JE, Blasier RB, Carpenter JE. Fractures of the acromion process: a proposed classification system. J Orthop Trauma. 1994;8:6–13.
18. Ogawa K, Naniwa T. Fractures of the acromion and the lateral scapular spine. J Shoulder Elb Surg. 1997;6:544–8.
19. Levy JC, Anderson C, Samson A. Classification of postoperative acromial fractures following reverse shoulder arthroplasty. J Bone Joint Surg Am. 2013;95(e104):1–7.

Chapter 3
Non-operative Management of Scapular Fractures: Patient Selection, Treatment Protocol, and Expected Outcomes

Robinson Esteves Pires, Pedro José Labronici, and Vincenzo Giordano

3.1 Patient Selection

The treatment of scapula fractures has substantially changed in the last decade. Although the scapula has a privileged muscular envelope which uneventfully heals the majority of fractures, scapular malunion and nonunion may significantly impair the shoulder girdle function, causing aesthetic deformities, impingement, chronic pain, and scapulothoracic dyskinesis (Fig. 3.1) [1].

The literature is controversial regarding the relative and absolute indications of operative management of scapular fractures. Although there are currently some recommendations for the surgical treatment of scapula fractures, there is still a sparse level of evidence to support them at a very high level [2–4].

Based on the patient characteristics, such as age, arm dominance, previous function, and occupation, the relative operative indications are the following:

- Articular displacement or gap >4 mm
- Articular involvement >20 to 25%
- Glenopolar (GP) angle ≤22°
- Translation of the scapula >20 mm (reduced to 10 mm for double disruptions and 15 mm when combined with 30° angulation)
- Angulation ≥45°

R. E. Pires (✉)
Department of the Locomotor Apparatus, Federal University of Minas Gerais, Belo Horizonte, Minas Gerais, Brazil

P. J. Labronici
Department of General and Specialized Surgery, Fluminense Federal University, Niterói, Brazil

V. Giordano
Orthopedics Department, Hospital Municipal Miguel Couto, Rio de Janeiro, Brazil

© The Author(s), under exclusive license to Springer Nature Switzerland AG 2024
R. E. Pires et al. (eds.), *Fractures of the Scapula*,
https://doi.org/10.1007/978-3-031-58498-5_3

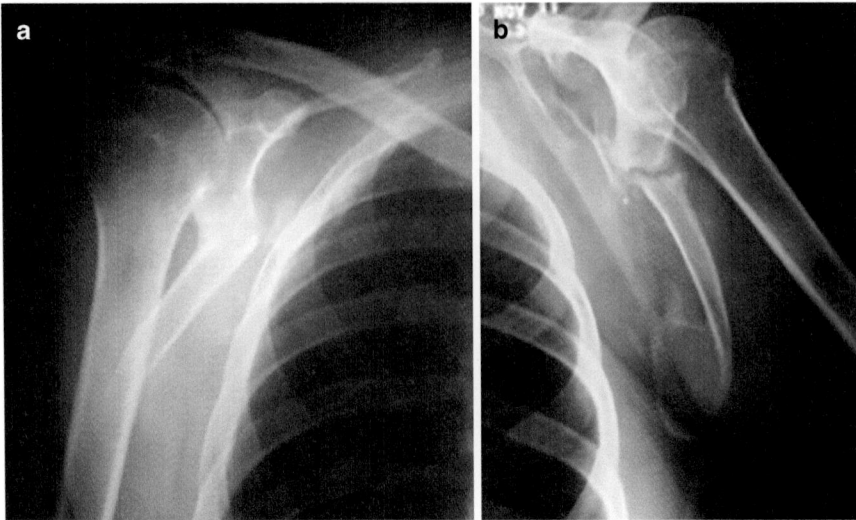

Fig. 3.1 (**a**) AP radiograph of the shoulder girdle of a 57-year-old male patient, demonstrating a malunion of the scapular body. Note the 90° rotation of the distal part of the body of the scapula relative to the proximal part of this bone. (**b**) Y radiographic view of the shoulder of a 45-year-old male patient, showing a nonunion of the scapular body

Careful evaluation of the GP angle should be performed to avoid misinterpretation of the correct measurement. A GP angle ranging from 30° to 45° is considered normal [1]. However, Labronici et al. [4] recommended that, whenever possible, measurement of GP angle should be taken in neutral rotation, since rotation of the scapula can either increase or decrease the measurement, therefore leading to a possible non-ideal indication for fracture fixation. The concept of medialization of the scapula also deserves to be analyzed with caution. Although the term medialization is universally used, Zuckerman et al. [5] advocate that lateral displacement of the glenoid with respect to the midline is a common finding in association with scapular fractures. This finding calls into question the commonly held belief that the predominant pattern of glenoid displacement is medial.

Another potential indication for surgical management of scapular fractures is the so-called floating flail chest, the association of ipsilateral floating shoulder and flail chest. Cunningham et al. [6] reported that the restoration of the scapula-clavicular arch, caused by the fixation of both clavicle and scapula fractures, unloads of the flail chest and improves pain control, respiratory function, thereby decreasing the duration of mechanical ventilation days and intensive care unit length of stay.

Indications for operative treatment of fractures in the elderly population must be carefully considered. Sometimes fixation of a scapula fracture may take hours with the patient resting in a semi-prone or prone position, leading to potential clinical complications, mainly regarding lung function, since the association scapula and rib fractures are relatively frequent. Bartonicek et al. [7] recommended to take into consideration not only the fracture pattern, but also the general clinical condition of the patient.

3.2 Treatment Protocol

The first description regarding scapula fractures may be found in the studies of French surgeons of sixteenth through eighteenth century. Ambroise Paré described a scapular fracture probably caused by war injury in 1579 [8, 9]. Then, Desault described the fracture of acromion and the fracture of the inferior angle of the scapula. His description also contained an original drawing of the Desault (apud Cole [10] and Bartonicek [11]) bandage designed by the author for management of the clavicle and scapula fractures (Fig. 3.2).

Our treatment protocol for non-operative management of scapular fractures consists initially of pain control and immobilization with a sling, followed by physical

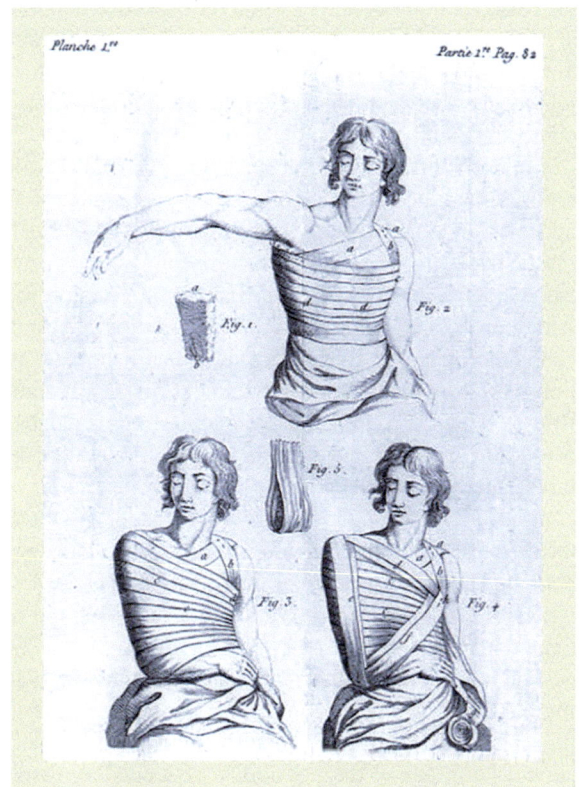

Fig. 3.2 Illustration of the original drawing of Desault bandage

therapy. Passive-assisted exercises start after pain control (usually after 14 days). Active-assisted exercises start after 21 days, according to the patient tolerance. Active exercises are initiated after 28 days [1]. A thoroughly detailed physiotherapy treatment protocol can be found in Chap. 13.

3.3 Expected Outcomes

The non-operative management of scapular fractures leads to favorable outcomes for most patients with scapular fractures [1]. Isolated non-displaced scapular body and glenoid neck fractures, as well as almost all acromion, coracoid process, and scapular spine fractures are adequately managed non-operatively [12]. In a systematic review of 520 scapula fractures, Zlowodzki et al. [12] found that 99% of all isolated scapula body fractures and 83% of all glenoid neck fractures were treated non-operatively, with excellent or good outcomes achieved in up to 86% and 77% of the cases, respectively. However, the authors observed that 80% of all glenoid fossa fractures were managed operatively, with excellent or good results in 82% of the cases. Schofer et al. [13], in a retrospective cohort study of 51 patients with an average follow-up of 65 months, also reported favorable functional outcomes after non-operative management of scapula fractures. Kim et al. [14] reported a positive relationship between smaller GP angle and poor Constant-Murley functional outcome in patients with floating shoulders.

Vander Voort et al. [15], in a database of 10,097 patients with scapular fractures, reported that the incidence of operative treatment of scapula fractures was 1.96% and 2.84% for open reduction and internal fixation (ORIF) and total shoulder arthroplasty, respectively. Scapular fractures previously treated with open reduction internal fixation were at significant risk for conversion to total shoulder arthroplasty. Although open reduction and internal fixation of scapular fractures did not significantly increase over time, both total or hemi-shoulder arthroplasty and overall (fixation + arthroplasty) operative treatment of scapula fractures increased significantly from 2007 to 2015. Functional outcomes of this database were not reported.

Although we completely agree that non-operative management of scapular fractures generally lead to favorable outcomes, the findings of the study by Vander Voort et al. [15] reporting that only 1.96% of patients with scapular fractures underwent ORIF must be interpreted with caution, since most studies report that 12–20% of patients benefit from surgical treatment [1]. Figure 3.3 shows the case of a patient who suffered a scapular body fracture involving the base of the coracoid process treated non-operatively.

Fractures of the inferior angle of the scapula have currently gaining attention in the literature. Although non-displaced or minimally displaced inferior angle fractures can be safely managed non-operatively, with favorable reported outcomes, one should be aware of the possibility of secondary displacement due to the muscle forces that act over the inferior angle on the scapula. The non-operative management of displaced inferior angle fractures can lead to malunion or nonunion,

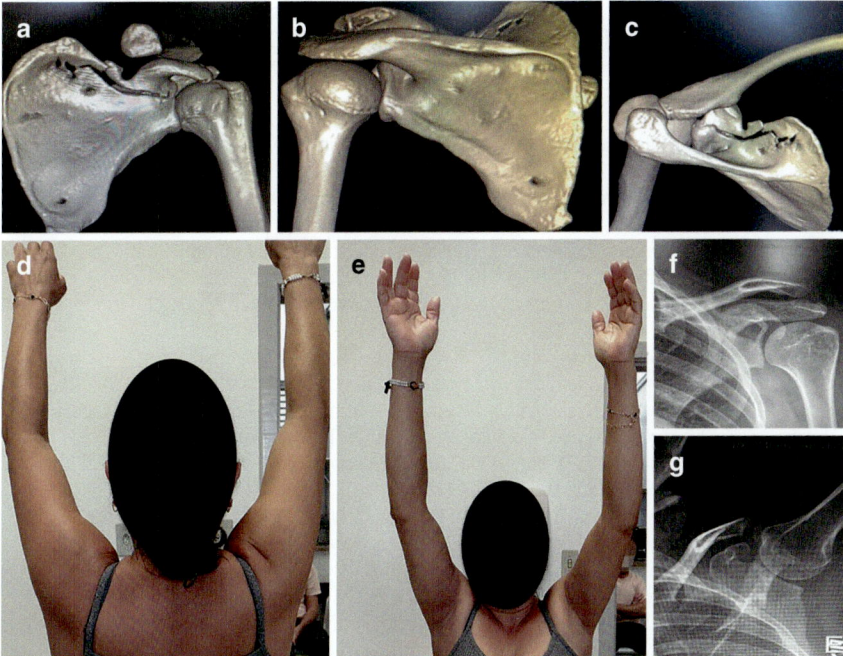

Fig. 3.3 A 32-year-old female patient suffered a motorcycle accident and presented a minimally displaced coracoid basis fracture that was non-operatively managed. (**a–c**): 3D CT scan showing the minimally displaced coracoid basis fracture. (**d** and **e**): Clinical aspect after fracture healing. Observe the almost complete range of motion of the left shoulder. (**f** and **g**): Radiographs after complete fracture healing

potentially generating a pseudo-winging scapula [16]. Although scapula fractures of the inferior angle, particularly with oblique lines oriented from medial proximal to lateral distal, are very rare, Min et al. [17] believe that such fracture pattern would be regarded as an avulsion fracture of the serratus anterior muscle, thus requiring surgery.

References

1. Pires RE, Giordano V, Mendes de Souza FS, Labronici PJ. Current challenges and controversies in the management of scapular fractures: a review. Patient Saf Surg. 2021;15(6):1–18.
2. Bartoníček J, Tuček M. Infraglenoid fracture of the scapular neck fact or myth? Rozhl Chir. 2019;98(7):273–6.
3. Mayo KA, Benirschke SK, Mast JW. Displaced fractures of the glenoid fossa. Results of open reduction and internal fixation. Clin Orthop Relat Res. 1998;347:122–30.
4. Labronici PJ, Tavares AK, Canhoto EC, Giordano V, Pires RES, Silva LHP, Mathias MB, Rosa IM. Does the position of the scapula in relation to the glenopolar angle change the preferred treatment of extra-articular fractures? Injury. 2017;48(Suppl 4):S21–6.

5. Zuckerman SL, Song Y, Obremskey WT. Understanding the concept of medialization in scapula fractures. J Orthop Trauma. 2012;26:350–9.
6. Bartoníček J, Tuček M, Naňka O. Scapular fractures. In: Textbook of shoulder surgery. 1st ed. Cham: Springer Nature; 2019. p. 55–73.
7. Cunningham BP, Bosch L, Swanson D, McLemore R, Rhorer AS, Parikh HR, et al. The floating flail chest: acute management of an injury combination of the floating shoulder and flail chest. J Orthop Trauma Rehab. 2020;27(1):10–5.
8. Paré A. Les oeuvres d'Ambroise Paré, conseiller, et premier chirurgien du Roy. Paris: Gabriel Buon; 1579. p. VCV.
9. Peltier LF. Compound fracture of leg, Paré's personal care. Clin Orthop. 1983;178:3–6.
10. Cole PA. Scapula fractures. Orthop Clin N Amer. 2002;33:1–18.
11. Bartonícek J, Cronier P. History of the treatment of scapula fractures. Arch Orthop Trauma Surg. 2010;130:83–92.
12. Zlowodzki M, Bhandari M, Zelle BA, Kregor PJ, Cole PA. Treatment of scapula fractures: systematic review of 520 fractures in 22 case series. J Orthop Trauma. 2006;20(3):230–3.
13. Schofer MD, Sehrt AC, Timmesfeld N, Störmer S, Kortmann HR. Fractures of the scapula: long-term results after conservative treatment. Arch Orthop Trauma Surg. 2009;129(11):1511–9.
14. Kim KC, Rhee KJ, Shin HD, Yang JY. Can the glenopolar angle be used to predict outcome and treatment of the floating shoulder? J Trauma. 2008;64(1):174–8.
15. Vander Voort W, Wilkinson B, Bedard N, Hendrickson N, Willey M. The operative treatment of scapula fractures: an analysis of 10,097 patients. Iowa Orthop J. 2022;42(1):213–6.
16. Alder-Price AC, Pilch W, Zhuang CB, McLean J, Bain GI. Inferior angle of scapula fractures: a retrospective case series. J Orthop Surg. 2020;30(1):1–5.
17. Min K-D, Hwang S-H, Cho A-H, Lee BI. Treatment of scapula fractures of the inferior angle causing pseudowinging scapula. J Korean Orthop Assoc. 2014;49(2):165–71.

Chapter 4
Scapular Fractures in Children and Adolescents

Robinson Esteves Pires, Pedro José Labronici, and Vincenzo Giordano

4.1　Epidemiology

The first description of a scapular fracture in children is credited to South, in 1839, who published a case treated by Arnott, in 1838. Arnott recorded a scapular fracture in a 6-year-old boy who died after a fall from the tree. Autopsy showed fractures of the coracoid base and clavicle [1, 2].

Scapular fractures are mighty rare injuries in the immature skeleton patient, accounting for less than 1% of all fractures in children and adolescents. They occur more frequently in male than female patients, but the peak incidence occurs in the adolescence. The most common mechanism of injury is direct trauma, such as a fall or a blow to the shoulder [3–5]. Sports activities with direct trauma over the shoulder, such as bicycle, skateboard, and rollerblades can also result in scapular fractures [6]. Domestic violence is another potential source of scapular fractures in children and adolescents. Indirect trauma, such as a fall on an outstretched hand, can also result in scapular fractures [3–6].

Bartoníček and Naňka [2], in a review of the literature including 70 scapular fractures in children and adolescents, reported that the most frequent fracture pattern occurred in the coracoid process (26 patients with 13.5 years in average). In 11 cases, acromioclavicular injury was associated. Scapular body fractures occurred in 19 patients, with average age of 10.5 years. Inferior angle fractures of the scapula

R. E. Pires (✉)
Department of the Locomotor Apparatus, Federal University of Minas Gerais, Belo Horizonte, Minas Gerais, Brazil

P. J. Labronici
Department of General and Specialized Surgery, Fluminense Federal University, Niterói, Brazil

V. Giordano
Orthopedics Department, Hospital Municipal Miguel Couto, Rio de Janeiro, Brazil

© The Author(s), under exclusive license to Springer Nature Switzerland AG 2024
R. E. Pires et al. (eds.), *Fractures of the Scapula*, https://doi.org/10.1007/978-3-031-58498-5_4

were found in 11 patients. Fractures of the acromion occurred only in four patients, with a mean age of 14.5 years. Glenoid fractures, more specifically avulsion of the distal two-thirds of the glenoid fossa, were identified in only three patients. Finally, scapulothoracic dissociation was observed in five patients, with a mean age of 13 years.

4.2 Diagnosis

The diagnosis of scapular fractures can be challenging, especially in the context of domestic violence. Specifically in these population, especially if fractures of the posterior costal ribs are seen on radiographic images, it is essential to suspect the existence of an associated fracture of the scapula, which is considered highly specific for child abuse [7].

The clinical presentation may vary depending on the energy of trauma and type, severity, and location of the fracture. Common signs and symptoms include pain, edema, and limited range of motion of the traumatized shoulder.

Imaging work-up is essential in the diagnosis of scapular fractures in children and adolescents. Radiographs are the initial imaging modality, but it can be insufficient to clearly show the fracture, particularly in non-displaced and minimally displaced fracture patterns. If there is a high index of suspicion for a scapular fracture, computed tomography (CT) scan may be necessary. Magnetic resonance imaging can be useful for identifying associated injuries, especially regarding soft tissues, but is not routinely used in the diagnosis of scapular fractures in children due to cost-related issues and need of sedation in such population. However, Alaia et al. [8], in 2017, based on a case series of eight patients, highlighted the importance of magnetic resonance imaging for diagnosis of an injury to the physis of the coracoid base.

4.3 Treatment

Treatment of scapular fractures in children and adolescents depends on the fracture type, location, degree of displacement, and the severity of trauma. Non-displaced or minimally displaced fractures can be safely managed non-operatively with rest, immobilization, and pain control. With the progression of the healing process (usually 2–3 weeks), the rehabilitation process is started. Displaced fractures or fractures associated with other injuries usually require operation [9, 10]. Operative management of scapular fractures in children and adolescents may include open reduction and internal fixation (ORIF) using screws or combined mini-fragment plates and screws. Fracture reduction with limited skin incision and percutaneous fixation is another option, depending on the fracture location and degree of displacement. ORIF is typically reserved for displaced fractures or fractures associated with other injuries. Bartoniček and Naňka [2] reported that operative management of scapular fractures was performed in five coracoid fractures associated with acromioclavicular dislocation, in three fractures of the inferior angle and in five cases of scapulothoracic dissociation.

Figures 4.1, 4.2, 4.3 and 4.4 depict a case of a 12-year-old boy who suffered a motorcycle accident and presented a blunt chest trauma with associated rib fractures, hemothorax, medial-third clavicle fracture on the right side, and a displaced fracture of base of the coracoid process, with associated acromioclavicular dislocation.

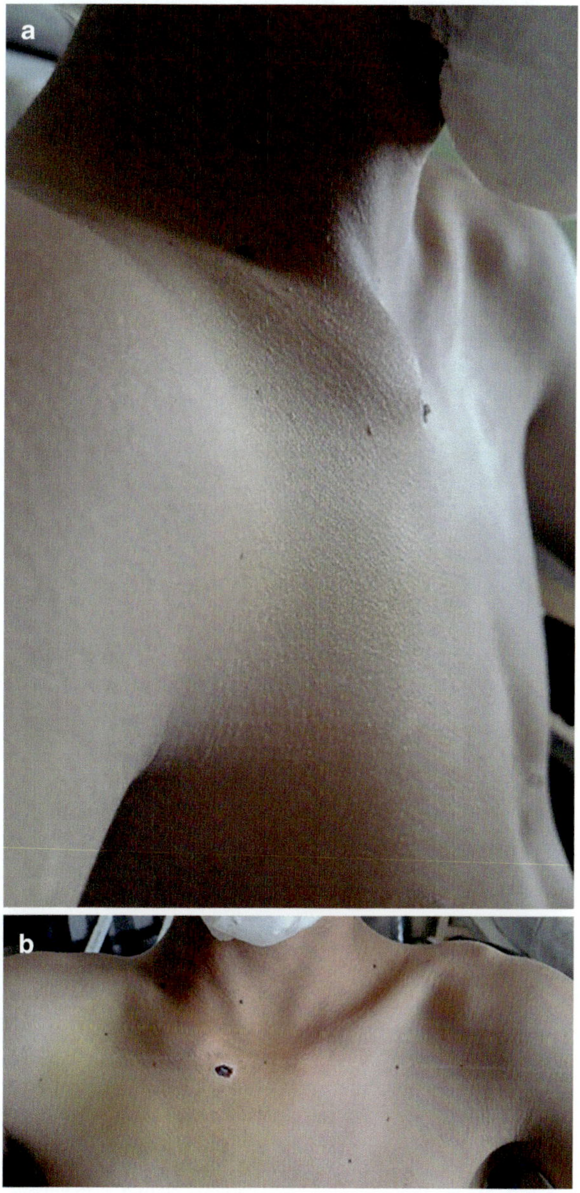

Fig. 4.1 Observe the clinical deformity on the right shoulder caused by the medial-third displaced clavicle fracture (**a**). On the left shoulder, observe the clinical deformity caused by the acromioclavicular dislocation (**b**)

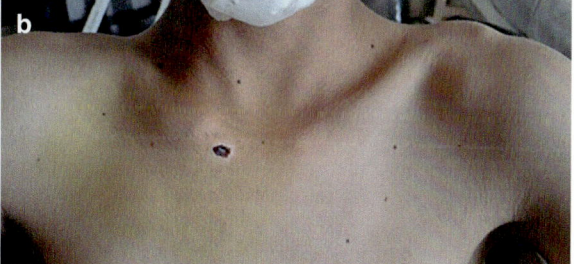

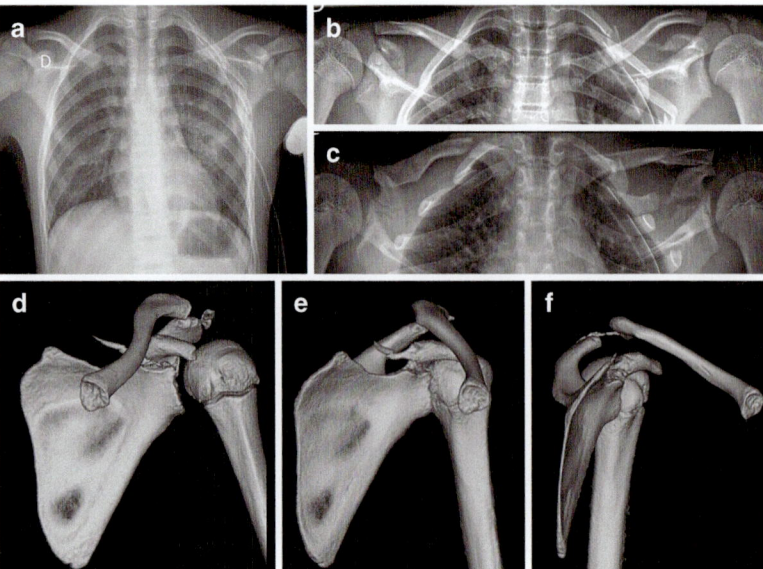

Fig. 4.2 Radiographs of the chest (**a**) and acromioclavicular joints (**b** and **c**) showing the rib fractures, medial-third clavicle fracture (right shoulder), and coracoid base fracture with associated acromioclavicular dislocation (left shoulder). (**d–f**) CT scan with 3D reconstruction details the coracoid base fracture with associated acromioclavicular dislocation

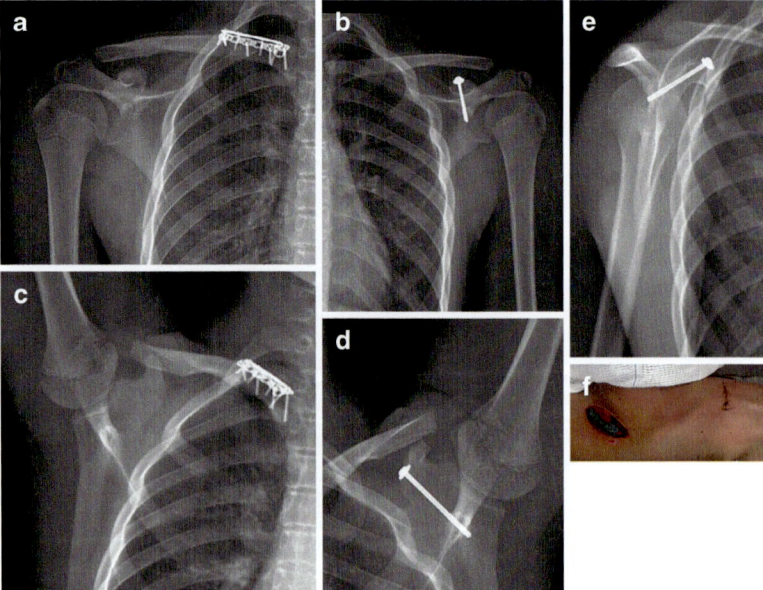

Fig. 4.3 Radiographs of the right and left shoulders showing complete fracture healing of both fractures. Observe the fixation of the clavicle fracture with double plating (2.4 mm variable angle plates) and fixation of the coracoid process with a 3.5 mm partially threaded screw (**a–e**). Note the reduction of the acromioclavicular joint. Intraoperative photograph showing the limited approach for coracoid process fixation and the double plating of the clavicle (**f**)

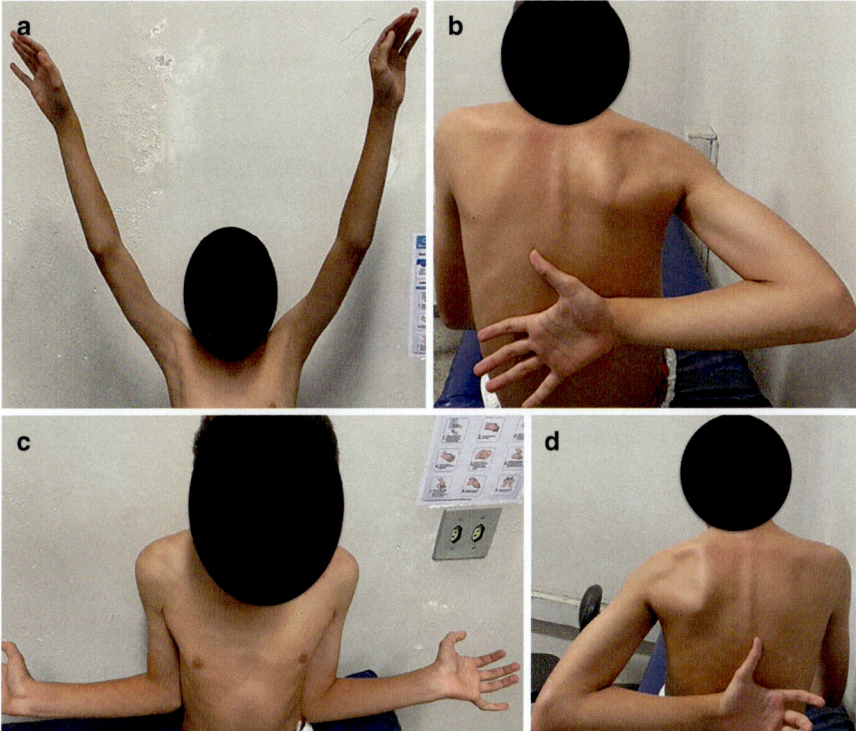

Fig. 4.4 Clinical aspect and range of motion of both shoulders after complete fracture healing (2 months post-op) (**a–d**)

4.4 Complications

Complications associated with scapular fractures in children and adolescents are also extremely rare. The vast majority of cases evolve with satisfactory functional recovery. However, in unrecognized or delayed treated fractures, complications such as nonunion, malunion, and chronic pain may occur. In addition, scapular fractures can be associated with other injuries, such as rib fractures, pneumothorax, acromioclavicular injuries, or brachial plexus injuries that require appropriate and individualized care. Finally, one should suspect of child abuse when a scapular fracture is observed in this population.

References

1. South JF. Case of fracture of the coracoid process of the scapula with partial dislocation of the humerus forwards and fracture of the acromion process of the clavicle. Med Chir Trans. 1839;22:100–9.
2. Bartoniček J, Naňka O. History of diagnostics and treatment of scapular fractures in children and adolescents and its clinical importance. Arch Orthop Trauma Surg. 2022;142:1067–74.

3. Bae DS. Scapular fractures in children and adolescents. J Pediatr Orthop. 2012;32(Suppl 1):S64–8.
4. Cantrell WC, Rineer CA, Jahangir AA, Taves C, Orr S, Casillas M. Scapular fractures: incidence, mechanisms, and outcomes. J Trauma. 2010;69(3):533–7.
5. Hennrikus W, Shah SA, Mooney JF, Schoenecker PL. Scapular fractures in children and adolescents. J Pediatr Orthop. 1996;16(2):157–61.
6. Albert MC, Ahmad CS. Scapular fractures. In: Makhmalbaf H, Makhmalbaf H, editors. Pediatric and adolescent sports injuries. Cham: Springer; 2020. p. 429–38.
7. Walker A, Kepron C, Milroy CM. Are there hallmarks of child abuse? I. Osseous injuries. Acad Forensic Pathol. 2016;6(4):568–90.
8. Alaia EF, Zehava Sadka Rosenberg ZS, Rossi I, Zember J, Roedl JB, Pinkney L, Steinbach LS. Growth plate injury at the base of the coracoid: MRI features. Skeletal Radiol. 2017;46:1507–12.
9. Mehlman CT, Crawford AH, McMillion TL, Roy DR. Operative treatment of adolescent scapular body fractures. J Pediatr Orthop. 1998;18(3):332–7.
10. Mueller M, Nazarian S, Koch P, Schatzker J. Scapular fractures in children and adolescents: a review of the literature and case report. J Pediatr Orthop. 1994;14(4):478–84.

Chapter 5
Approaches and Fixation Strategies for Scapular Fractures (Pitfalls and Opportunities): MIO Versus Conventional ORIF

Nathaniel E. Schaffer, Jaclyn M. Kapilow, and William T. Obremskey

5.1 Approaches

All posterior approaches, including the original Judet and its modifications, can be performed in either the lateral decubitus or prone positions. When a concomitant anterior approach is required, either for an anterior glenoid fracture or an ipsilateral clavicle fracture, the lateral position may be preferred to permit both approaches without repositioning. Prone positioning may be preferred to ease retraction with a Judet-style incision or to improve glenoid exposure with the shoulder resting in an abducted and externally rotated position. Anterior approaches may be performed in the lateral, supine, or beach-chair positions. Imaging should be obtained prior to draping to ensure that the necessary Grashey and scapular-Y views can be obtained (Fig. 5.1).

5.1.1 Judet and Modifications

5.1.1.1 Posterior Exposure of the Scapular Body ("Judet")

The posterior approach to the scapula, or Judet approach, is useful for complex scapular fractures involving the posterior glenoid, the lateral and medial borders of the scapula, and the scapular spine as it provides access to all posterior surfaces of the bone. It is particularly useful for fractures that are difficult to mobilize or reduce due to late presentation, malunion, or requiring direct manipulation of multiple

---

N. E. Schaffer · J. M. Kapilow · W. T. Obremskey (✉)
Division of Orthopaedic Trauma, Vanderbilt University Medical Center, Nashville, TN, USA

© The Author(s), under exclusive license to Springer Nature Switzerland AG 2024
R. E. Pires et al. (eds.), *Fractures of the Scapula*,
https://doi.org/10.1007/978-3-031-58498-5_5

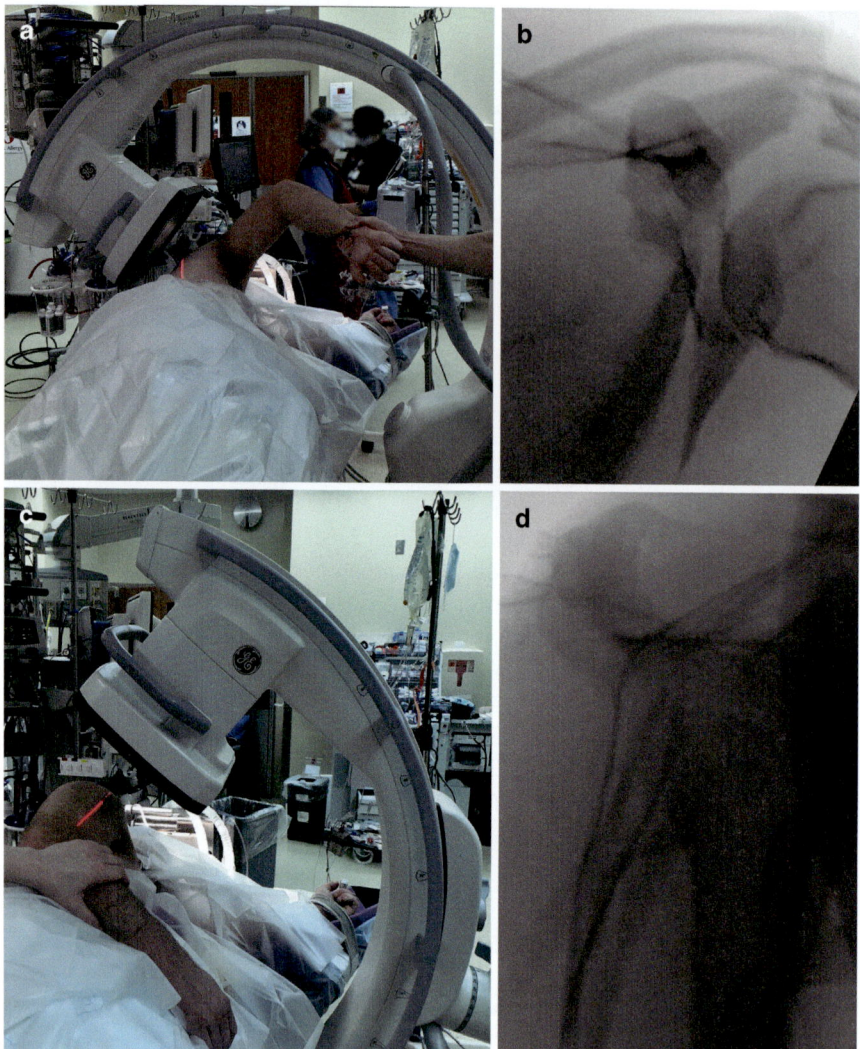

Fig. 5.1 (**a**, **b**) In the lateral position, the Grashey view. (**c**, **d**) The scapular-Y view

fragments. Although the approach elevates a large portion of the posterior musculature from the scapular body, perfusion to the bone is maintained by the anterior musculature, which remains undisturbed.

The patient is positioned prone or lateral with the ipsilateral arm draped into the field. An incision is made from the lateral border of the acromion along the scapular spine and down the medial subcutaneous border of the scapula to the inferior angle (Fig 5.2a). Electrocautery is then used to elevate the deltoid origin off the scapular spine and the infraspinatus origin off the medial border, leaving a small cuff of tissue for later repair. The entire musculo-fasciocutaneous flap is then elevated

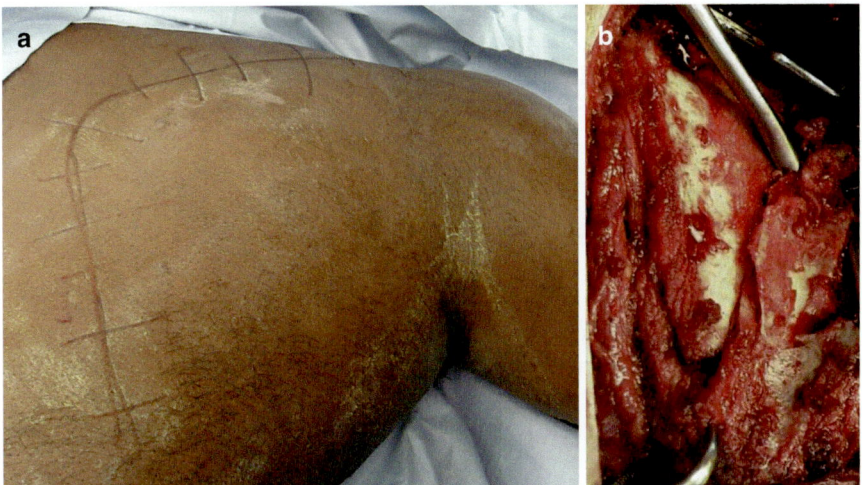

Fig. 5.2 (**a**) In the classic Judet approach, the incision is made along the scapular spine and medial border. (**b**) A full-thickness skin flap can be elevated laterally

laterally to expose the entire dorsal surface of the scapula (Fig 5.2b) [1]. Alternatively, a full-thickness skin flap can be elevated first so that the deltoid and infraspinatus can be elevated independently from each other. If the latter method is used, dissection is carried sharply to the fascia, and a cutaneous flap is raised off the fascia past the lateral border of the scapula using heavy scissors. Electrocautery is used to control bleeding from vessels perforating the fascia. It is critical to elevate all the subcutaneous tissue off the fascia as part of the flap. Spreading the tissue with heavy scissors helps define this plane. Dissection with cautery decreases initial bleeding but makes the plane more difficult to differentiate. The fascia along the inferomedial border of the deltoid is incised, and the posterior deltoid is released sharply from the scapular spine and reflected laterally [2, 3]. A suture placed in the medial aspect of the deltoid fascia facilitates retraction during dissection. The infraspinatus is released sharply from the medial border of the scapula. Subperiosteal dissection of the infraspinatus is then carried laterally to expose the scapular body to its lateral border. Especially when performed as originally described, this approach can limit visualization of the glenoid.

Care must be taken to protect the suprascapular neurovascular bundle as it emerges from the spinoglenoid notch. The neurovascular pedicle limits the extent of lateral retraction, and during dissection it is at greatest risk in the triangle formed by the spinoglenoid notch, a point 4 cm medial to the notch along the scapular spine, and a point 7 cm caudal to the notch along the lateral border of the scapula where the circumflex scapular artery emerges [4]. The ascending branch of the circumflex scapular artery may need to be ligated, but it also can be transected by the fracture and may resume bleeding during dissection. We recommend having medium vascular clips readily available. Following reduction and fixation, the infraspinatus is reattached medially to the rhomboid fascia using non-absorbable suture. Repair through bone tunnels in the medial scapula is also possible. Similarly, the deltoid can be reattached with non-absorbable suture to a fascial cuff or through drill tunnels to the scapular spine. Subcutaneous drains may be used to help reduce the risk of postoperative seroma [2].

5.1.1.2 Infraspinatus Sparing ("Modified Judet")

Because much of the central body of the scapula is quite thin, fixation is typically achieved along the periphery of the bone, and as such, most of the bony surface revealed by elevating the infraspinatus is not useful for fixation. Therefore, a modified approach may be used in which a skin flap is raised as described above but the infraspinatus is left in place. After retracting the deltoid and exposing the scapular spine, the intermuscular and internervous interval between the infraspinatus (supraspinatus nerve) and teres minor (axillary nerve) is developed taking care to identify and ligate the ascending branch of the circumflex scapular artery, which is found approximately 3 cm caudal to the glenoid along the lateral margin of the scapula and can retract anteriorly causing significant blood loss if avulsed [4]. Both muscles are contained in a single fascial compartment, which can obfuscate the plane between them. Elevating the fascia reveals the tripinnate infraspinatus medial and cranial to the unipennate teres minor [3]. The lateral pillar of the scapula is found between them and is used for reduction and fixation (Fig. 5.3a). If needed, a separate deep window can be made with sharp dissection through the fascia to the subcutaneous

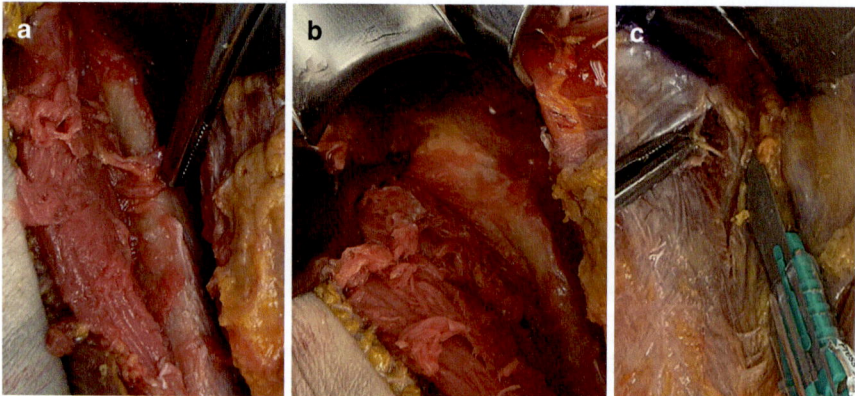

Fig. 5.3 The medial and lateral plating surfaces can be exposed without releasing the deltoid or elevating the entirety of the infraspinatus. (**a**) The plane between the infraspinatus and teres minor is developed to reveal the lateral pillar of the scapula and the circumflex scapular artery as it emerges posteriorly. (**b**) Retraction of both the deltoid and the infraspinatus without releasing either muscle. (**c**) Dissection along the spine and medial border of the scapula reveals the medial plating surface

medial border of the scapula where plates can also be placed (Fig. 5.3c) [2]. A plate may also be placed on the exposed scapular spine if needed. Although this modified exposure provides access to only 17% of the bony surface exposed in the classic approach, the primary fixation surfaces remain available [5].

5.1.1.3 Deltoid Sparing

As a further modification of the Judet approach, the posterior deltoid may be retracted superolaterally instead of releasing its origin from the scapular spine. The same deep interval between the infraspinatus and teres minor is then exploited to visualize the lateral scapular body (Fig 5.3b). Although this modification reduces the extent of medial visualization at the base of the scapular spine, it still exposes 91% of the surface exposed by the modified Judet approach [6]. As such, the deltoid may be left intact in the vast majority of fractures and reflected only if the glenoid neck fracture extends superiorly and the patient is obese or extremely muscular.

5.1.1.4 Infraspinatus Tenotomy

When direct reduction of an intra-articular glenoid fracture is required through a glenohumeral arthrotomy, visualization of the glenoid surface can be difficult, even with a distractor placed on Schanz pins in the scapular spine and the bare area of the proximal humerus. To enhance exposure, the infraspinatus tendon can be divided sharply 1 cm medial to its insertion on the greater tuberosity and reflected laterally. When performed in the prone position, this release increases the exposure from 63% to 97% of the glenoid articular surface (Fig. 5.4a) [7]. To date, the effect on clinical outcome from this release and the resultant improved exposure is unknown.

5.1.1.5 Triceps Release

Improvement of the exposure provided by the posterior approach has been described by releasing the origin of the long head of the triceps brachii from the inferior neck of the glenoid. Although the clinical effects of this release are not well described in the literature, the release has been reported to increase the bony surface exposed by 13%, particularly along the inferior glenoid neck, and it permits palpation of the anterior glenoid (Fig. 5.4b). Therefore, releasing the triceps may be helpful when reducing and fixing certain fractures involving the glenoid [5].

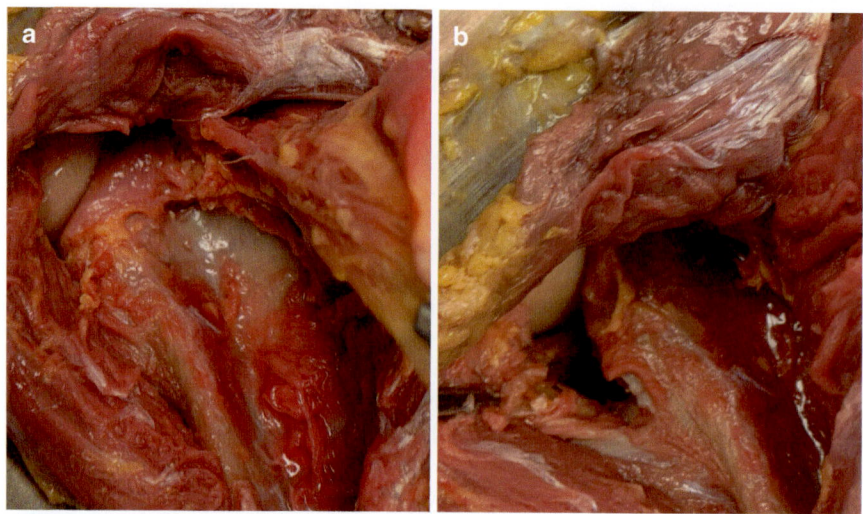

Fig. 5.4 (**a**) Tenotomy of the infraspinatus improves exposure of the glenoid. (**b**) Triceps tenotomy can improve exposure of the inferolateral glenoid and permit palpation of the anterior articular surface

5.1.2 Reverse Judet

The "Reverse Judet" approach uses the same deep dissection as other posterior approaches but with a skin flap that is based medially rather than laterally. A skin incision is made along the scapular spine to the lateral border of the acromion before curving caudally and distally along the lateral border of the scapula (Fig. 5.5). A full-thickness flap is elevated, and deep dissection proceeds as previously described above. This incision may be preferred for surgical fixation of the glenoid and the lateral scapular body [3].

5.1.3 Lateral Window and Minimally Invasive

To limit the risk of postoperative seroma, it is feasible in some cases to make separate incisions directly over the areas where surgical fixation will be performed. One incision is made along the lateral border of the scapula and glenoid, and through this lateral window, the previously described deep dissection is developed by retracting the deltoid and exposing the lateral border of the scapula in the plane between the infraspinatus and teres minor muscles. A second incision is often required to expose the medial or caudal exit of the major fracture line. Commonly, this incision is medial and parallel to the first extending from the medial scapular spine along the

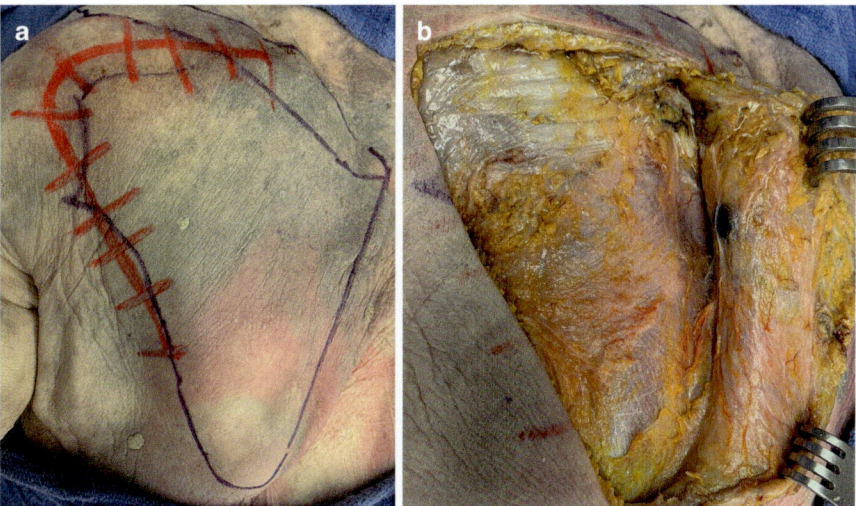

Fig. 5.5 (**a**) The skin incision for the "Reverse Judet" approach curves from the lateral border of the scapula along the scapular spine. (**b**) A full-thickness skin flap is elevated medially

medial border of the scapular body. Dissection is then carried sharply onto the subcutaneous medial surface of the scapula permitting exposure of that common fracture exit site. Plating from the vertebral border of the scapula onto the scapular spine can be performed through this window. However, because fracture patterns vary, the location of the second incision should be tailored to the fracture. Dissection can be performed sharply to the subcutaneous border of the scapula anywhere along the scapular spine or medial border, and the second skin incision should be placed directly over the intended plating surface [8].

5.1.4 Deltopectoral

Although most scapular fractures are approached posteriorly, fractures of the anterior glenoid or coracoid are best addressed anteriorly, and the deltopectoral approach to the shoulder, familiar to many surgeons, may be used [9]. The patient is positioned supine on a radiolucent table or in the beach-chair position with a bump under the medial border of the scapula. The ipsilateral arm and shoulder are draped into the field. An incision is made from the lateral clavicle directly over the coracoid and along the medial aspect of the anterior deltoid. Only the superior extent of the incision is required for isolated coracoid fractures [10]. The cephalic vein is identified and protected in the interval between the deltoid and pectoralis major muscles, which is developed bluntly after sharp dissection through the investing fascia. The subscapularis is released by tenotomy or osteotomy of the lesser tuberosity, depending on the surgeon's preferred method of later repair, and reflected medially to expose the anterior glenoid. Care should be taken to avoid avulsing the anterior circumflex humeral artery and its *venae comitantes* as they enter the field at the caudal aspect of the subscapularis tendon. If improved visualization of the glenoid neck is required, the coracoid may be osteotomized and repaired at the end of the operation [9, 11]. Some fractures requiring a posterior approach also have an anterior articular fragment attached to the coracoid. In these cases, a small approach in the proximal aspect of the deltopectoral interval with the patient in the lateral position permits direct manipulation of the coracoid and attached articular surface.

5.2 Fixation Strategies

5.2.1 *Reduction*

After exposing the relevant fracture lines, they are mobilized to permit reduction. In the case of delayed presentation, abundant callus may need to be debrided, and a lamina spreader may be required. Reduction of body fractures typically begins by medializing the laterally displaced body to the glenoid fragment, working simultaneously on the medial and lateral borders simultaneously when necessary [2, 12]. A shoulder hook or *kugelspitz* (applied in a 2-mm pilot hole) in the laterally displaced body fragment can provide adequate control, or a towel clip or small pointed-reduction clamp may be used to grasp and move the lateral body fragment medially to the glenoid. When the lateral border is aligned, Kirschner wires provide provisional fixation. The reduction can be adjusted using modified pointed-reduction clamps applied through pilot holes. Alternatively, a plate-assisted reduction may be accomplished with a short plate applied across the fracture line along the lateral border [2]. When necessary, a 4-mm Schanz pin in the scapular neck can serve as a joystick and may be used for provisional fixation by applying an external fixator between it and a pin in the body [12]. After restoring alignment of the scapular body and neck, separate glenoid fragments can be reduced to it using similar techniques.

Anterior coracoid and glenoid rim fractures are a challenge to reduce and stabilize. Lateral positioning can hinder visualization. If the posterior rim is intact, the articular surface can be visualized by releasing the subscapularis and levering the humerus posteriorly with a retractor placed on the posterior rim of the glenoid. Releasing the coracobracialis tendon or osteotomizing the tip of the coracoid can also improve visualization. Coracoid fragments along with any attached articular surface can be positioned by direct manipulation or by inserting a Schanz pin into the base of the coracoid. Fluoroscopic rather than direct reduction may be necessary.

5.2.2 Fixation

As a flat bone, the scapula is as thin as 3 mm in its central portion thickening to 8–10 mm along the lateral border and spine and 25 mm at the glenoid vault [13]. Because of this, fixation is typically placed along the margins and 2.7- or 2.4-mm plates are typically preferred over 3.5-mm plates. With the need to place such short screws, locking technology may be advantageous [14]. Along the medial border, a 2.7- or 2.4-mm reconstruction plate (typically 12-holes in length) can be contoured to curve up onto the caudal surface of the scapular spine (Fig. 5.6). Pediatric Kocher clamps may be used to produce the required contour [12]. A 2.7-mm locking compression plate provides a rigid option with locking holes, but a reconstruction plate may be preferred to permit extension of this plate onto the posterior surface of the glenoid when needed. A French bender is useful to generate the necessary plate contour (Fig. 5.6). Independent screws may also be necessary to secure intra-articular glenoid fractures, and buttress plates along the inferomedial glenoid neck can also helpful [9]. Finally, when necessary, independent 2.7- or 3.5-mm cortical screws or cannulated screws may be placed from anterior to posterior or vice versa in the coracoid (Fig. 5.6). Anteriorly, the start point must be on the medial side of the coracoid to keep the screw intra-osseous, and care should be taken to avoid breaching into the supraspinatus fossa.

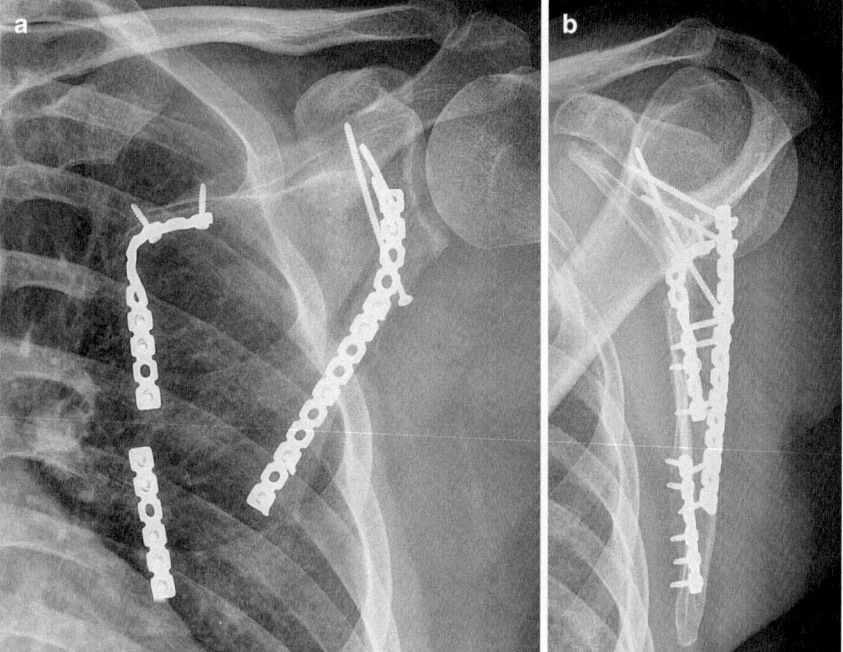

Fig. 5.6 (**a**) Grashey and (**b**) scapular-Y radiographic views of a typical fixation construct

5.3 Advantages and Drawbacks of Minimally Invasive Approaches

Minimally invasive approaches improve functional outcome scores, decrease blood loss, and lower risk of wound infection [15]. Additionally, minimally invasive approaches preserve more muscular attachments and may permit earlier motion. With delayed presentation, debridement of callus from all fracture lines may require a classic Judet approach.

5.4 Summary

Most scapula fractures are best approached posteriorly. Skin incisions may be made directly over the spine or medial or lateral borders, or a full-thickness skin flap may be elevated from medial to lateral or lateral to medial. The deltoid may be retracted or reflected off the scapular spine. Reduction and fixation are primarily performed along the thicker pillars of bone on the inferolateral and medial borders of the infraspinatus as well as along the scapular spine. Although most of the footprint of the infraspinatus on the scapular body can typically be preserved, the muscle can be reflected when necessary. For difficult fractures with delayed presentation, a full-thickness musculo-fasciocutaneous flap may be elevated from medial to lateral as originally described by Judet. When needed, the deltopectoral approach provides anterior exposure. Fixation typically comprises 2.7-mm or 2.4-mm plates.

References

1. Judet R. Traitement chirurgical des fractures de l'omoplate. Acta Orthop Belg. 1964;30:673–8.
2. Obremskey WT, Lyman JR. A modified judet approach to the scapula. J Orthop Trauma. 2004;18(10):696–9.
3. Ebraheim NA, Mekhail AO, Padanilum TG, Yeasting RA. Anatomic considerations for a modified posterior approach to the scapula. Clin Orthop. 1997;334:136–43.
4. Wijdicks CA, Armitage BM, Anavian J, Schroder LK, Cole PA. Vulnerable neurovasculature with a posterior approach to the scapula. Clin Orthop. 2009;467(8):2011–7.
5. Harmer LS, Phelps KD, Crickard CV, Sample KM, Andrews EB, Hamid N, et al. A comparison of exposure between the classic and modified Judet approaches to the scapula. J Orthop Trauma. 2016;30(5):235–9.
6. Salassa TE, Hill BW, Cole PA. Quantitative comparison of exposure for the posterior Judet approach to the scapula with and without deltoid takedown. J Shoulder Elb Surg. 2014;23(11):1747–52.
7. Garlich JM, Samuel K, Nelson TJ, Monfiston C, Kremen T, Metzger MF, et al. Infraspinatus tenotomy improves glenoid visualization with the modified Judet approach. J Orthop Trauma. 2020;34(3):158–62.
8. Gauger EM, Cole PA. Surgical technique: a minimally invasive approach to scapula neck and body fractures. Clin Orthop. 2011;469(12):3390–9.

9. Hardegger FH, Simpson LA, Weber BG. The operative treatment of scapular fractures. J Bone Joint Surg Br. 1984;66(5):725–31.
10. Hill BW, Jacobson AR, Anavian J, Cole PA. Surgical management of coracoid fractures: technical tricks and clinical experience. J Orthop Trauma. 2014;28(5):e114–22.
11. Hoppenfeld S, De Boer PG, Buckley R. Surgical exposures in orthopaedics: the anatomic approach. 4th ed. Philadelphia: Wolters Kluwer/Lippincott Williams & Wilkins Health; 2009.
12. Cole PA, Dubin JR, Freeman G. Operative techniques in the management of scapular fractures. Orthop Clin North Am. 2013;44(3):331–43, viii
13. Burke CS, Roberts CS, Nyland JA, Radmacher PG, Acland RD, Voor MJ. Scapular thickness—implications for fracture fixation. J Shoulder Elb Surg. 2006;15(5):645–8.
14. Cole PA, Gauger EM, Schroder LK. Management of scapular fractures. J Am Acad Orthop Surg. 2012;20(3):130–41.
15. Jiang B, Lu J, Kang X, Li L, Jiang S, Gong X. Minimally invasive surgery for complex scapular fractures through small incisions combined with titanium miniplate fixation. Int J Clin Exp Med. 2016;9(9):18124–32.

Chapter 6
Special Considerations: Fractures of the Scapular Neck and Body

Kyle Auger, Jaclyn M. Jankowski, Richard S. Yoon, and Robinson Esteves Pires

6.1 Introduction

Fractures of the scapular neck and body commonly occur secondary to high energy trauma [1]. They have been shown to be associated with concomitant injuries, commonly rib and clavicle fractures [2]. As with any injury, a decision should be made on whether to pursue non-operative versus operative management based on fracture tolerances and patient factors. When it comes to scapular neck and body fractures specifically, there have been several studies looking at various types of approaches and fixation strategies, and the outcome of each technique.

6.2 Operative Approaches

Classically, the workhorse approach used for fixation of scapula fractures is the Judet approach. The Judet approach is the most comprehensive, and when done properly, can expose the entire scapula to allow for reduction maneuvers and definitive fixation. As discussed in previous chapters, the Judet approach starts with a large boomerang skin incision along the scapular spine and medial border

---

K. Auger · J. M. Jankowski · R. S. Yoon (✉)
Division of Orthopaedic Trauma & Adult Reconstruction, Department of Orthopaedic Surgery, Cooperman Barnabas Medical Center - RWJBH, Livingston, NJ, USA

Division of Orthopaedic Trauma & Adult Reconstruction, Department of Orthopaedic Surgery, Jersey City Medical Center - RWJBH, Jersey City, NJ, USA

R. E. Pires
Department of the Locomotor Apparatus, Federal University of Minas Gerais, Belo Horizonte, Minas Gerais, Brazil

© The Author(s), under exclusive license to Springer Nature Switzerland AG 2024
R. E. Pires et al. (eds.), *Fractures of the Scapula*,
https://doi.org/10.1007/978-3-031-58498-5_6

producing a flap. Next, the origin of the deltoid muscle is dissected off, and the infraspinatus is mobilized and reflected [3]. It is important to note that for most orthopaedic surgeons, operative scapula fractures are a rare entity; therefore, the authors must recommend that for most operative scapula fractures, the Judet approach should be the mainstay, workhorse approach. Unless you are at a tertiary referral center for these types of injuries, the minimally invasive approaches that are subsequently described should be reserved for higher volume surgeons.

The original description of the Judet approach included the take down of the posterior deltoid in order to help provide exposure to the scapula. Historically, this extensive approach has a high rate of iatrogenic complications and can lead to slower recovery post-operatively [3]. Salassa et al. [4] performed a cadaveric study that quantified the amount of posterior scapula that could be exposed during the Judet approach with takedown of the posterior deltoid muscle versus without takedown of the posterior deltoid muscle. It was found that an average of 30.2 cm^2 vs 27.3 cm^2 of the scapula could be exposed with or without deltoid takedown, respectively, which was found to be statistically significant. This correlates to the deltoid sparing approach allowing for exposure of 91% of the bony scapula. In all specimens, the limited approach gave access to vital points of fixation including the posterior glenoid, spinoglenoid notch, and lateral scapula border. Many post-operative restrictions can be avoided if the insertions of the posterior deltoid and infraspinatus muscles are maintained. The authors therefore recommend proceeding with complete takedown of the deltoid only if additional exposure is needed.

Graafland et al. [5] published a case series that included 74 patients who had either a displaced scapular body or neck fracture. Forty of these patients were treated surgically while 34 were treated conservatively with a majority of the surgically treated patients sustaining intraarticular fractures. Those undergoing surgical fixation were treated utilizing a Judet approach with or without takedown of the posterior deltoid. Their results demonstrated no significant difference between the two cohorts in terms of mean DASH scores (14.7 in surgical group and 9.8 in nonoperative group) or quality of life. A difference was seen in time to union within the surgical group depending on a technical difference. The patients that underwent a deltoid release had a time to union of 49 weeks versus 23 weeks in the patients who underwent a deltoid sparing procedure.

Utilizing the same skin incision as the Judet approach, Obremskey and Lyman described a modified Judet approach that utilizes the interval between the infraspinatus and teres minor musculature [6]. Figure 6.1 shows a cadaveric representation of the exposure obtained with this approach. They showed that limiting the muscular dissection decreased trauma to the rotator cuff musculature and protected the major neurologic structures, while still providing adequate exposure to the fracture. Costa et al. performed a cadaveric study specifically looking at the safety parameters of the major neurovascular structures during the modified Judet [7] approach. The group utilized the infraglenoid tubercle as the anatomic landmark between the cadavers to determine the distance between it and the axillary nerve and

6 Special Considerations: Fractures of the Scapular Neck and Body   47

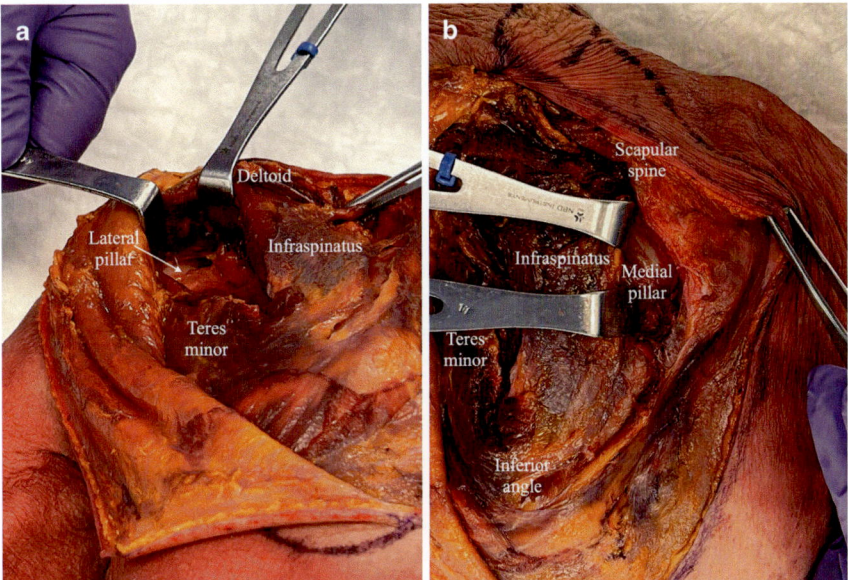

Fig. 6.1 Dissection of cadaver specimen demonstrating the interval for the modified Judet approach and exposure that can be obtained across the entire scapula. (**a**) shows the lateral pillar exposure, and (**b**) shows the medial pillar exposure

suprascapular nerve. These nerves are at high risk during this extensile approach. It was found that the average distance from the infraglenoid tubercle and the axillary nerve was 23.8 mm and the average distance for the suprascapular nerve was 33.2 mm. The study showed that this approach can provide safe access to fractures of the scapular neck and body.

An additional minimally invasive approach to scapular neck and body fractures has been described by Gauger and Cole [8]. This approach utilizes two small incisions that are made based on the site where the fracture exits on the perimeter of the scapula. With this technique, one can flip back and forth between incisions to sequentially reduce fracture fragments. By visualizing the distal edges of the fracture lines, direct reduction of the fracture can be obtained despite the minimal dissection. The approach is best utilized for simple fracture patterns that have singular exit points through the lateral and medial pillar. It is most successful if the fracture is being addressed acutely when the fragments are the most mobile.

A different approach can be utilized in simple fracture patterns especially in fractures that are either isolated to the lateral pillar or has a minimally displaced medial pillar that does not need reduction. Brodsky [9] originally described an approach utilizing a straight longitudinal incision to expose the lateral border of the scapula. It also utilizes the interval between teres minor and the infraspinatus. This approach can be beneficial in the setting of scapula fractures with displaced acromion fractures as well as the longitudinal incision can be extended proximally to allow proper exposure for appropriate fixation of the acromion.

6.3 Strategies for Fixation

Determining how to approach reducing fractures of the scapular neck and body largely is determined by the characteristics of the specific fracture pattern. If both the medial and lateral pillars are disrupted, it has been recommended that the most displaced column be addressed first for reduction [10]. More often than not, this tends to be the lateral column. Commonly a modified Judet is used or a minimally invasive approach that allows the ability to simultaneously address both pillars. Again, for most surgeons, the Judet or the modified Judet remains the workhorse approach to gain the most access, and when done appropriately, can lead to great outcomes, with minimal complications. When it comes to order of fixation, generally the medial pillar is secured with a more flexible implant first to create a hinge to assist in manipulating and final fixation of the lateral pillar. Use of a variety of reduction tools can allow for easier manipulation of individual fragments. Schanz pins can be placed into fragments for assistance with traction of the piece to help

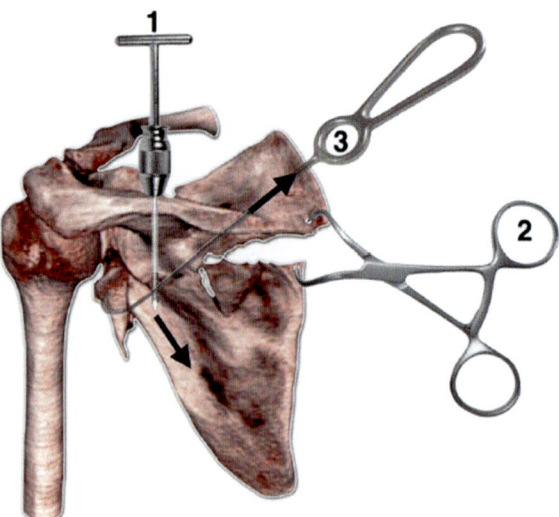

Fig. 6.2 Illustration demonstrating potential reduction sequence for a displaced fracture of glenoid and body of scapula exiting the medial pillar. (*1*) Schanz pin placed in body of scapula with traction in the caudal direction to correct the length of the lateral pillar. (*2*) A 2.5 mm drill is used to place two holes on each side of the medial pillar in order to utilize a pointed reduction clamp to reduce the medial column. (*3*) A bone hook is placed on the glenoid fragment and pulled to reduce the fragment. (*4*) Provisional K-wires can then be placed or mini fragment plates may be used to maintain reduction

correct length. A 2.5 mm drill bit can be utilized to place pilot holes in positions of fragments to place tines of a pointed reduction clamp in proper position perpendicular to fracture lines to compress together and hold reduction. Another useful tool is the bone hook, which can be used to hook the fragments on the edges of the pillars and bring them into position for proper reduction. Figure 6.2 gives an example of the sequence of reduction of a fracture of the scapula body and glenoid utilizing the various reduction methods just mentioned.

After achieving reduction of fracture fragments, the next important step is determining what fixation strategy is most appropriate for the best outcome. There are several companies that have created pre-contoured scapular body and neck plates. These are not necessarily always available or the most suitable option depending on fracture characteristics. One consideration that should be made is determining the amount of rigidity in the construct that one is creating. When addressing glenoid fractures where direct reduction is necessary for improved functional outcomes, a more rigid construct with locking options or compression plating should be considered. Construct rigidity should also be taken into consideration when initially fixating the medial or lateral pillars. A more flexible construct may be necessary in order to allow further reduction of fragments on the opposite pillar before final fixation is performed. A combination of 3.5 or 2.8 mm locking vs non-locking compression plates or reconstruction plates could be used and custom contoured to the patient's anatomy in order to create a unique construct per patient. If more flexibility is warranted, then the addition of 2.4 and 2.0 mini fragment plates can be added for increased flexibility.

Burke et al. [11] performed cadaveric studies looking at the thickness of the scapula and the impact this could have on fracture fixation. What they showed was that the thickest parts of the scapula are the glenoid fossa, the lateral border of the scapula, and the scapular spine. The thickness was shown to be 25, 9.7, and 8.3 mm, respectively. Something of importance to note is that the average thickness in the central portion of the scapular body was found only to be 3 mm. This should be taken into consideration when trying to obtain the best purchase for fracture fixation. If amenable, the surgeon should attempt to utilize the thicker portions of the scapula which include the lateral border and the scapular spine for the best screw purchase for implant fixation. With scapular neck fractures in mind specifically, a mechanical study by Sulkar et al. [12] looked at different fracture fixation constructs utilizing either single plate on the lateral column or dual parallel plating. After cyclic loading of the constructs, displacement was smaller and column stiffness was higher with the dual parallel plating technique. These differences were found to be small but were significant.

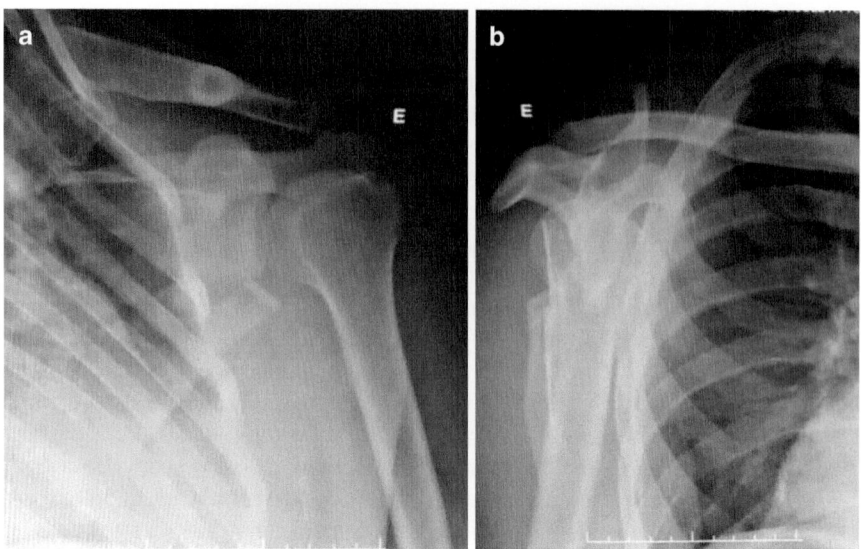

Fig. 6.3 Left shoulder radiographs of a 34-year-male patient who was involved in motorcycle accident demonstrating a significantly displaced scapular neck fracture with extension into the scapular body. (**a**) Grashey view and (**b**) scapular Y view

6.4 Case Example: A 34-Year-Male after a Motorcycle Crash

A 34-year-male presents to the trauma bay following a motorcycle crash. This is a closed injury, and the patient is neurovascularly intact. Preoperative work-up and radiographs indicate scapular neck and body fracture with increased glenopolar angle (GPA) of 20° and excessive medialization greater than 20 mm (Figs. 6.3a, b and 6.4a–f).

Here, the patient was positioned in the lateral decubitus position with the chest tilting slightly anterior. The ipsilateral arm was placed in 90° from the chest and properly padded. The C-arm was brought in from the posterior aspect of the patient. The C-arm was then rainbowed over the patient with the detector on the posterior aspect of the patient and the collimator on the anterior aspect. Finally, it was tilted toward the head of the patient to decrease interference with the surgeon. The C-arm positioning is shown in Fig. 6.5. Utilizing a bean bag can allow for more freedom of movement to also get the appropriate views of the glenohumeral joint as well.

The Judet approach was performed in order to fully expose the fracture fragments, and then fragment specific reduction and fixation were achieved.

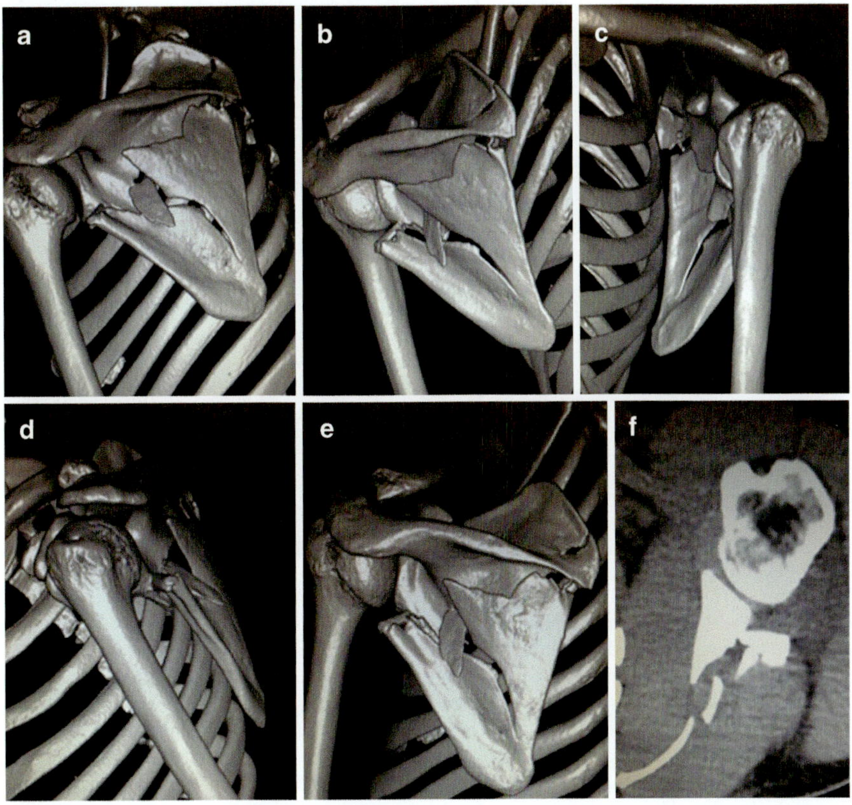

6 Special Considerations: Fractures of the Scapular Neck and Body 51

Fig. 6.4 (**a**)–(**e**) show 3D CT reformations of left shoulder of a 34-year-male patient involved in motorcycle accident. The reformations demonstrate the significant medialization of the glenoid with fracture lines involving the medial pillar and scapular body. (**f**) shows axial CT cut of the left shoulder demonstrating fracture of the scapula body and intraarticular glenoid fracture involving >25% of the articular surface

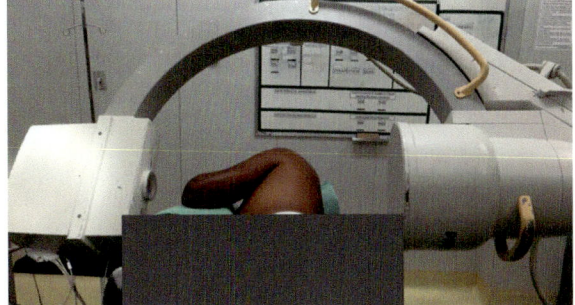

Fig. 6.5 Demonstration of position of C-arm while patient is in the lateral decubitus position to obtain quality X-rays during scapula fixation

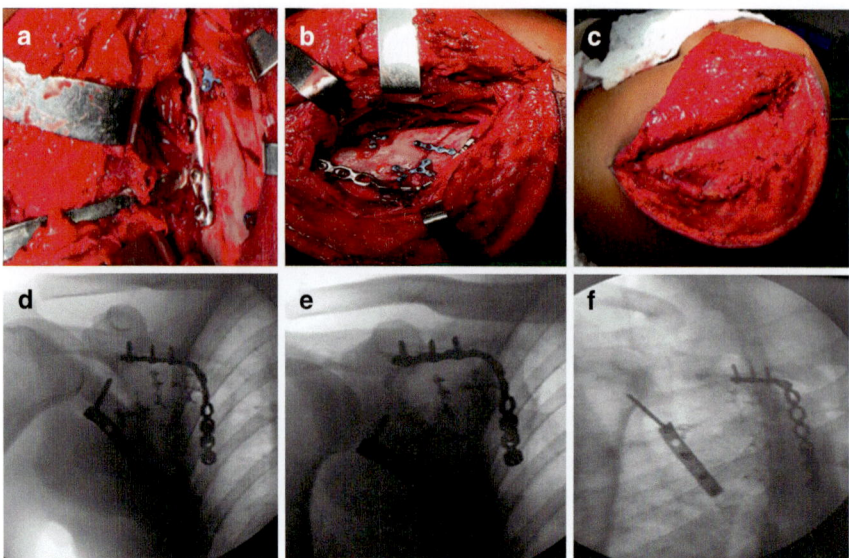

Fig. 6.6 (**a**)–(**c**) are the clinical images obtained from the case of the 34-year-male who was involved in the motorcycle accident. (**a**) shows the exposure and fixation used for the scapular neck and lateral pillar. It involved a combination of a one-third tubular plate in buttress mode and a mini fragment plate. (**b**) shows the exposure and fixation used for the medial pillar. It involved a combination of a reconstruction plate custom contoured to the patient's anatomy and various shaped mini fragment plates. (**c**) shows the deep closure of the muscular attachments back to their origins which completely covers the hardware that was used. (**d**)–(**f**) shows the intraoperative fluoroscopic images that were obtained after hardware placement demonstrating appropriate reduction and fixation of the fracture. The various views obtained also demonstrate that all screws are of appropriate length and are not prominent or intraarticular

Figure 6.6a–f show the clinical images of the exposure with fixation in place as well as the intraoperative images obtained demonstrating appropriate placement of hardware and reduction of fracture. Additional adjuncts, noted in Fig. 6.2, provide examples of reduction aides that can be extremely helpful prior to definitive fixation, which in this case was provided by several mini and small fragment plates to

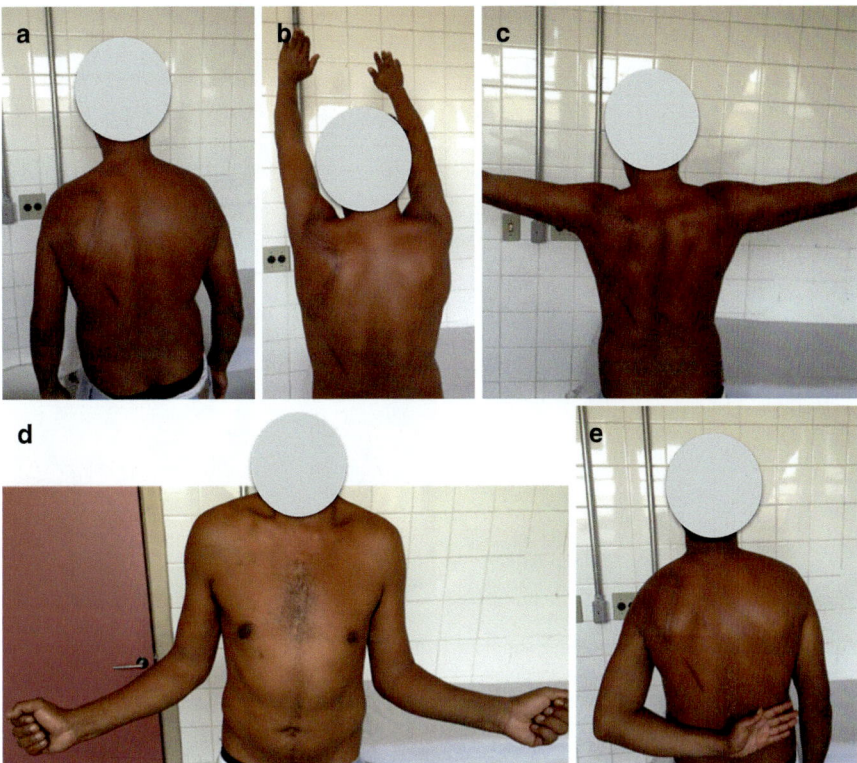

Fig. 6.7 Clinical photographs demonstrating patients range of motion at 8 weeks post-operatively from left scapula open reduction and internal fixation via a Judet approach. (**a**) demonstrates a well healed surgical incision. (**b**) demonstrates symmetric forward flexion. (**c**) demonstrates symmetric shoulder abduction. (**d**) demonstrates symmetric external rotation. (**e**) demonstrates internal rotation to L2

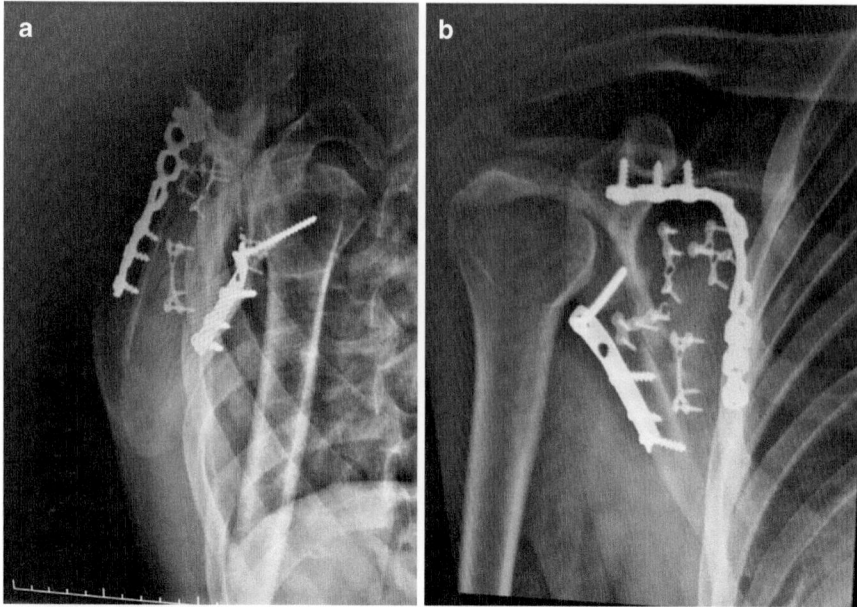

Fig. 6.8 Eight-week post-operative shoulder radiographs of a 34-year-male patient involved in motorcycle accident. (**a**) shows a scapular Y view, and (**b**) shows an AP of left shoulder demonstrating healed fracture of the scapula with no signs of hardware failure or loosening

restore and maintain the scapular anatomy. For closure, the muscular attachments are brought back to the origins and sutured down. In some cases, the deltoid origin can be repaired via bone tunnels. A deep drain was also placed to prevent hematoma. Post-operatively, active, active-assist range of motion was started immediately, with advancing to strengthening and passive range of motion at week 6 upon radiographic signs of healing. Figures 6.7a–e and 6.8a, b depict the patients' radiographic and clinical findings at 8 weeks which show this patient recovering well and ultimately, he went on to uneventful healing.

6.5 Summary

Approaching scapular neck and body fractures requires consideration of surgical approach, reduction technique, and fixation construct. If increased visualization of the scapula is needed, a Judet approach with deltoid sparing or a modified Judet approach can be utilized. For more simple fracture patterns, a minimally invasive approach can be used. In regard to reducing fracture fragments, the most displaced column should be addressed first and to aid the reduction one can utilize tools such as Schanz pins, pointed reduction clamps, and bone hooks. With respect to fixation constructs, utilizing a combination of reconstruction and compression plates custom contoured to the patient's anatomy allow unique constructs to address the specific fracture pattern. Having knowledge of these various approaches and tips will help produce quality outcomes in patients with surgically indicated scapular neck and body fractures.

References

1. Tuček M, Chochola A, Klika D, Bartoníček J. Epidemiology of scapular fractures. Acta Orthop Belg. 2017;83(1):8–15.
2. Lantry JM, Roberts CS, Giannoudis PV. Operative treatment of scapular fractures: a systematic review. Injury. 2008;39(3):271–83.
3. Bartoníček J, Tucek M, Lunácek L. Judetův zadní prístup k lopatce [Judet posterior approach to the scapula]. Acta Chir Orthop Traumatol Cechoslov. 2008;75(6):429–35.
4. Salassa TE, Hill BW, Cole PA. Quantitative comparison of exposure for the posterior Judet approach to the scapula with and without deltoid takedown. J Shoulder Elb Surg. 2014;23(11):1747–52.
5. Graafland M, van de Wall BJM, van Veelen NM, van Leeuwen R, Hoepelman RJ, Knobe M, et al. Long-term follow-up of patients with displaced scapular fractures managed surgically and non-operatively. Injury. 2022;53(6):2087–94.
6. Obremskey WT, Lyman JR. A modified Judet approach to the scapula. J Orthop Trauma. 2004;18(10):696–9.
7. da Costa MP, Braga AC, Geremias RA, Tenor Junior AC, Ribeiro FR, Brasil Filho R. Anatomy of the scapula applied to the posterior surgical approach: safety parameters during access to the lateral angle. Rev Bras Ortop (Sao Paulo). 2019;54(5):587–90.
8. Gauger EM, Cole PA. Surgical technique: a minimally invasive approach to scapula neck and body fractures. Clin Orthop Relat Res. 2011;469(12):3390–9.
9. Brodsky JW, Tullos HS, Gartsman GM. Simplified posterior approach to the shoulder joint. A technical note. J Bone Joint Surg Am. 1987;69(5):773–4.
10. Pires RE, Giordano V, de Souza FSM, Labronici PJ. Current challenges and controversies in the management of scapular fractures: a review. Patient Saf Surg. 2021;15(1):6.
11. Burke CS, Roberts CS, Nyland JA, Radmacher PG, Acland RD, Voor MJ. Scapular thickness—implications for fracture fixation. J Shoulder Elb Surg. 2006;15(5):645–8.
12. Sulkar HJ, Tashjian RZ, Chalmers PN, Henninger HB. Mechanical testing of scapular neck fracture fixation using a synthetic bone model. Clin Biomech (Bristol, Avon). 2019;61:64–9.

Chapter 7
Special Considerations: Articular Involvement (Glenoid Fossa and Rim)

Vincenzo Giordano, David Rojas, and Robinson Esteves Pires

7.1 Glenoid Fractures and Associated Injuries

The prevalence of scapular fractures has been documented as 1% of all bone fractures. Glenoid fractures contribute to 3–5% of all fractures around the shoulder and up to 10–20% of all scapular fractures [1–5]. Common concomitant orthopedic and non-orthopedic injuries linked to glenoid fractures are injuries to the lungs, head, brachial plexus, and/or peripheral nerves. Ipsilateral humeral and clavicle fractures are also representative, in addition to other injuries frequently seen in polytraumatized patients [1, 2, 4].

7.2 Anatomys

The glenoid fossa or cavity is a critical anatomical structure within the later aspect of the scapula (socket), supporting the humeral head and creating the GH joint, which functions as a diarthrodial and multiaxial joint. The stability of the GH joint is also contingent on other important static and dynamic anatomical restrains within the shoulder, providing stability and motion in multiple planes. The glenoid fossa is

---

V. Giordano (✉)
Orthopedics Department, Hospital Municipal Miguel Couto, Rio de Janeiro, Brazil

D. Rojas
Faculty of Medical Sciences Minas Gerais (FCMMG), Educational Foundation Lucas Machado (FELUMA), Belo Horizonte, Brazil

R. E. Pires
Department of the Locomotor Apparatus, Federal University of Minas Gerais, Belo Horizonte, Minas Gerais, Brazil

© The Author(s), under exclusive license to Springer Nature
Switzerland AG 2024
R. E. Pires et al. (eds.), *Fractures of the Scapula*,
https://doi.org/10.1007/978-3-031-58498-5_7

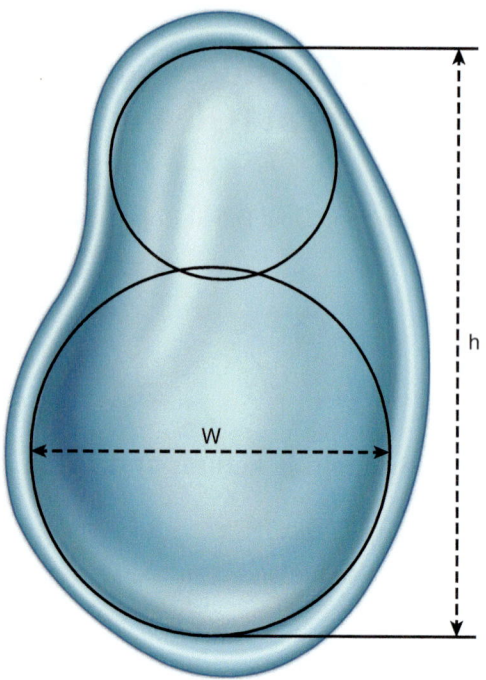

Fig. 7.1 Illustration of the glenoid fossa as a "pear shape" format with two overlapping circles

a shallow structure with a surface-area ratio of 4:1 when compared to the humeral head, warranting high levels of shoulder range of motion (ROM) [1]. Key static and dynamic stabilizing soft tissue restrain structures include the fibrocartilage brim, labrum, GH ligaments, rotator cuff, and capsule. These key anatomical restrains assist in joint support and functionality while preventing GH dislocations [1, 5]. Seidl et al. illustrated that the glenoid fossa as "pear-shaped" format were two circles with different radii overlap to each other (Fig. 7.1). The glenoid height and width on average measure ~32 and ~25 mm, respectively. However, these measurements are variable upon patients' sex and height [1, 6].

The glenoid fossa is slightly retroverted 1° in reference to the scapular axis and can present with a neutral variance up to 5° [1, 7]. The arterial supply of the glenoid is constituted by the suprascapular artery, anterior and posterior circumflex arteries in addition to perforating branches from the rotator cuff [1, 8].

7.3 Injury Mechanism

Fractures to the glenoid are commonly related to (1) direct lateral and high-energy impact injury mechanism to the shoulder, (2) indirect injury through axial loading with the arm in an outstretched position, or (3) in the settings of GH instability [1, 5, 9]. Over 90% of the glenoid fossa, neck and/or scapular body fractures are associated with high-energy trauma. Therefore, patients must always be thoroughly evaluated to assess for additional orthopedic and non-orthopedic injuries that could lead to detrimental results [1, 10, 11]. Patients with glenoid fractures in the settings of low-energy injury mechanism will frequently report a previous history of shoulder instability, sport-related trauma, or seizures resulting in shoulder dislocation [1, 3, 5]. These types of fractures generally distress the anterior or anteroinferior aspect of the rim, leading to avulsion fractures. Posterior shoulder dislocation may also be associated with posterior glenoid fossa and/or rim fractures, resulting in posterior shoulder instability [1, 12].

7.4 Diagnosis (Physical Examination and Imaging Workup)

A comprehensive physical examination is mandatory in all polytraumatized patients with suspected scapular fractures. In the "multiple injured patient", resuscitation and clinical stabilization are paramount before attention is placed to other non-emergent and secondary injuries. Immediately after polytraumatized patients are appropriately resuscitated and clinically stable, non-emergent orthopedic injuries should be evaluated and managed in a timely manner. In patients with extra-articular scapular and/or glenoid fractures, a detailed physical exam must be completed. Always start with inspection to look for any obvious deformity, open wounds, swelling, vascular status, active and passive ROM. Additionally, a detailed neurological exam must be performed since up to 10% of patients with glenoid fractures can present with neurological deficits, from either a brachial plexus and or peripheral nerve palsy [1, 4]. Finally, it is always important to consider patients' age, pre-injury functional level, as well as occupational goals and limb dominance. This helps surgeons guide decision-making process.

Essential radiographic workup includes anteroposterior (AP or true AP/Grashey), scapular Y and axillary views. Advanced imaging studies, such as Computerized Tomography (CT) scans with or without three-dimensional (3D) reconstruction are recommended for superior understanding of the glenoid anatomy and fracture patterns and rule out glenoid fractures that could have been missed on plain radiographs [1, 3, 5, 10]. Three-dimensional (3D) reconstruction CT scans have demonstrated to be critical for surgical planning and execution [1, 2, 10]. Magnetic resonance imaging (MRI) is not mandatory in the settings of acute fractures of the glenoid, although these are helpful when evaluating fractures in the setting of chronic instability or associated soft tissues injuries, such as rotator cuff pathology [1, 13].

7.5 Classification

The original Ideberg classification system of glenoid fractures continues to be wisely utilized among orthopedic surgeons, acknowledging it's low to moderate interobserver and intraobserver reliability ($R < 0.2$ and R 0.46), respectively [1, 14].

The Ideberg classification system underwent modifications from Goss et al. to include a total of six fracture configurations (Ideberg-Goss) [1, 4, 15]. The type (Ia) and (Ib) intra-articular or avulsion type fractures involve the anterior rim (Ia) or posterior rim (Ib), which are often related to GH dislocation events. The Ideberg-Goss fracture classification types II, III, and IV are intra-articular fractures and will present with a concomitant fracture line extension through the scapular neck, or complete body on type IV glenoid fractures. Type V glenoid fractures include those combinations or subtypes between Ideberg II, III, and IV glenoid fractures. Finally, type VI intra-articular glenoid fractures correspond to all comminuted fracture variations of the glenoid and scapular anatomy (Fig. 7.2) [4]. In 2013, the AO foundation proposed a new and more reliable classification system for glenoid fractures [1, 14, 16]. The AO classification system incorporates three main categories: F0, F1, and F2, and a sub-classification based on four anatomical quadrants of the glenoid (antero-superior, anteroinferior, postero-superior, postero-inferior). F0 illustrates all extra-articular or glenoid neck fractures. F1 types are those intra-articular fractures presenting with distinctive variations or subtypes. F1 subtypes include fracture to the anterior rim (F1.1) fracture to the posterior rim (F1.2), and (F1.3) are those transverse or short oblique intra-articular fractures. F2 configurations correspond to intra-articular and multifragmentary (≥3 fragments) fractures (F2.1), and those presenting with a central fracture dislocation are considered (F2.2 subtype) (Table 7.1 and Fig. 7.3) [1, 17]. Recently, Bartoníček et al. [18] developed a classification

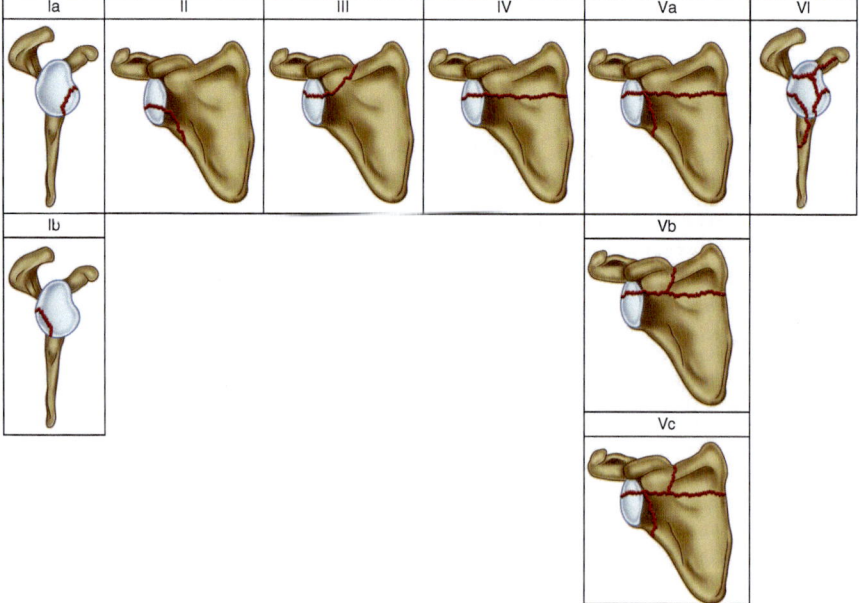

Fig. 7.2 Ideberg—Goss fracture classification of the scapula

7 Special Considerations: Articular Involvement (Glenoid Fossa and Rim)

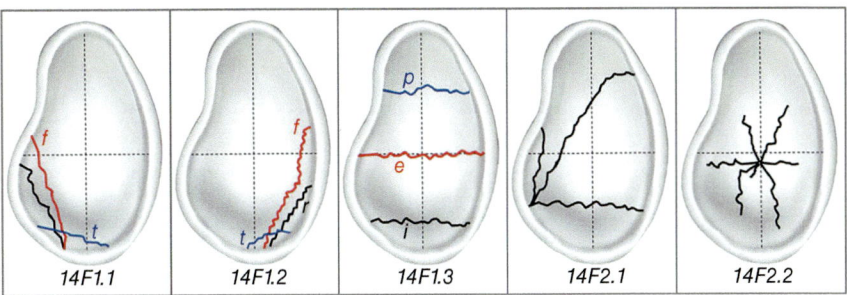

Fig. 7.3 The AO scapula fracture classification

Table 7.1 AO classification for glenoid fractures

Glenoid fracture	Subtype	Qualification
14F0, Extra-articular	Glenoid neck	
14F1, Simple, intra-articular	1.1: Anterior glenoid rim	f: Infraequatorial, single quadrant
	1.2: Posterior glenoid rim	r: Supraequatorial, 2 quadrants
		t: Infraequatorial, 2 quadrants
	1.3: Transverse/short oblique	i: Infraequatorial
		e: Equatorial
		p: Supraequatorial
14F2, Multifragmentary	2.1: ≥3 articular fragments	
	2.2: Central fracture-dislocation	
14B, Extension into body	1: Exits body at ≤2 points	
	2: Exit body at ≥3 points	

system based on 3D reconstruction CT scans, assessing fracture configurations while comparing them with intraoperative findings. This classification system differs from traditional classifications based solely on simple radiographic imaging. Therefore, it is of great utility for preoperative planning, in addition to its prognostic ability when compared to other classifications. Five fracture types or variations were described based on CT 3D reconstruction scans [superior glenoid (SG), anterior glenoid (AG), posterior glenoid (PG), inferior glenoid (IG) and the entire glenoid (EG)]. The superior glenoid (SG) fossa fractures are then divided into three subtypes determined by fragment size (type A, B, and C), and its fracture line extension to the upper border of the scapula. Type A are avulsion fractures measuring up to one quarter (<25%) of the glenoid fossa surface. Type B fractures present with a fragment size superior to a third (>33%) of the fossa. Type C fractures are those characterized by a split of half (50%) of the superior glenoid surface (Figs. 7.4 and 7.5).

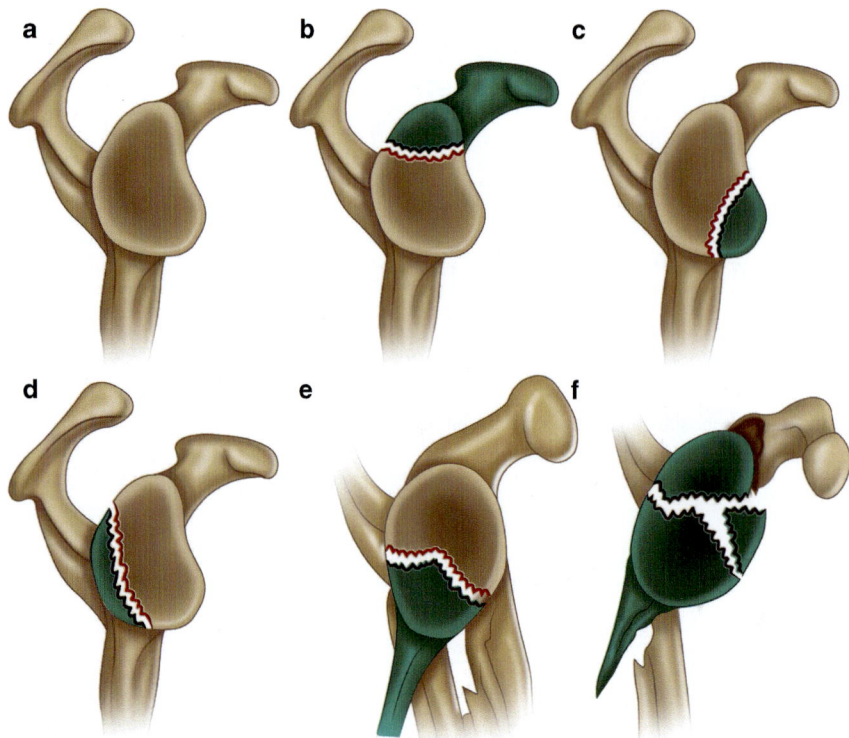

Fig. 7.4 Bartoníček fracture classification of the glenoid fossa. (**a**) Lateral view of the normal glenoid; (**b**) superior glenoid (SG) fracture; (**c**) anterior glenoid (AG) fracture; (**d**) posterior glenoid (PG) fracture; (**e**) inferior glenoid (IG) fracture; (**f**) entire glenoid (EG) fracture

Anterior glenoid (AG) fractures are also categorized by fragment size into three subtypes (peripheral, overhang, and vertical split). The "peripheral" rim fractures of the AG fall within the bony Bankart lesion. Avulsion of 25% the anteroinferior fragment is classified as an "overhang" subtype. The "vertical split" subtype entails any vertical tear crossing longitudinally through the glenoid, creating a two-piece separation of 30–50% of the total glenoid surface. Concerning posterior glenoid (PG) fractures, two main fracture subtypes were established (comminuted and single fragment). Inferior glenoid (IG) fractures include fragments of the distal inferior glenoid. These can present as non-displaced or displaced inferior fragments and are frequently associated with a fracture line extension from the inferior rim to the lateral scapular border or body. The fragment sizes are stratified as small, medium, or large and can be located within the distal quarter (25%), the distal third (33%), distal half (50%), and distal two thirds (60%) of the overall surface glenoid fossa. Three types of distal glenoid fracture lines are seen within this fracture configuration (transverse, oblique, and inverted V shape). Lastly, fractures of the entire glenoid

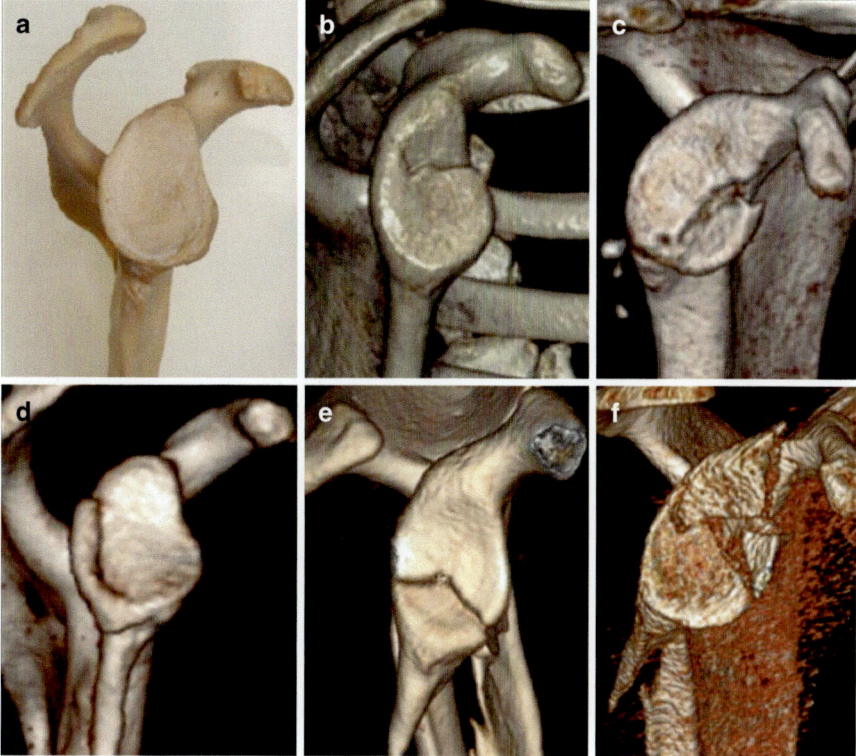

Fig. 7.5 Bartoníček fracture classification of the glenoid fossa CT scan reconstruction

(EG) fossa usually present with a complete fracture of the articular surface and an associated dissociation of the scapular neck and/or body [18].

7.6 Treatment of Glenoid Fossa and Rim Fractures

Management of glenoid fractures can be divided into two main groups: non-operative and operative treatment. When evaluating treatment options and strategies, it is essential to have a comprehensive understanding of the anatomy, fracture pattern and associated scapular fracture line extensions, as well as associated and concomitant orthopedic and non-orthopedic injuries. Moreover, it is essential to recognize patients' goals and expectations, which are fundamental for prognosis, recovery, and satisfaction. Generally, glenoid fractures presenting with over 20% of

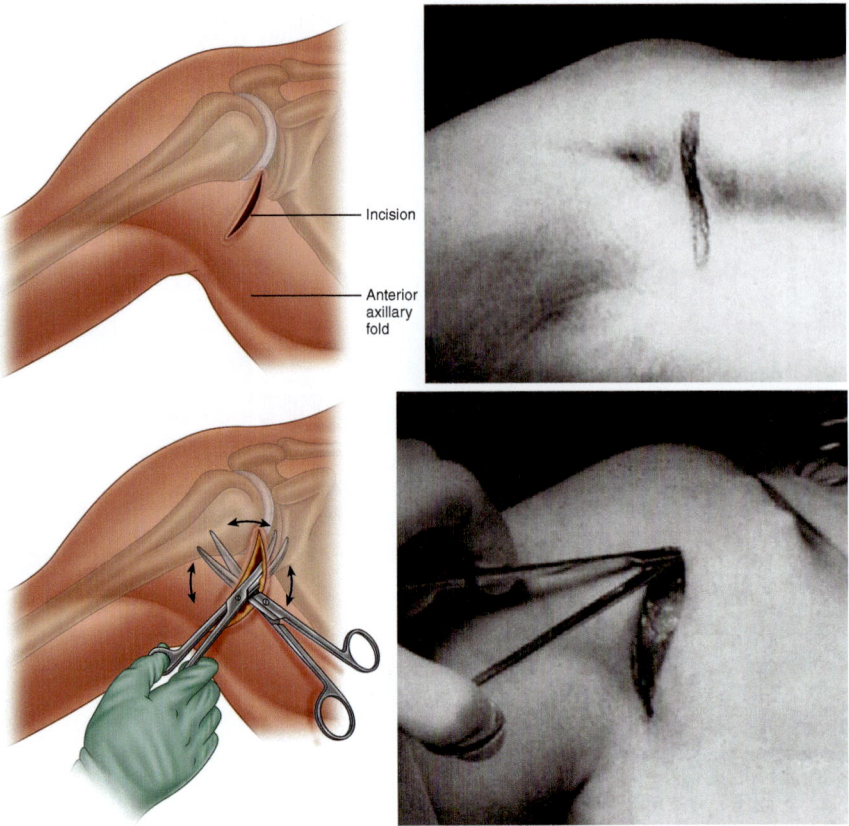

Fig. 7.6 Anterior axillary incision to approach the shoulder joint

articular surface involvement will require surgical treatment with open reduction and internal fixation (ORIF). Arthroscopically assisted fracture fixation associated with labrum repair is another treatment option, depending on the fragment size and fracture pattern. There is no consensus regarding a "tolerable" articular step-off guiding non-operative versus operative treatment. Certain authors have suggested a tolerable articular "step-off" ranging from 2 up to 10 mm; however, to this date no universal consensus exists [1, 19, 20]. The most common surgical approach for the treatment of intra-articular glenoid fractures is the deltopectoral approach. The anterior deltopectoral approach provides adequate visualization of the glenohumeral joint and articular surface, being an effective option for the management of anterior glenoid fossa and rim fractures. Leslie and Ryan have described the anterior vertical axillary approach for the treatment of fractures located in the anterior and anteroinferior glenoid. This anterior and small vertical axillary incision allows for appropriate exposure to the anterior and anteroinferior border of the glenoid without requiring an extensive dissection to the shoulder joint (Fig. 7.6) [21, 22].

7.6.1 Anterior Vertical Axillary Approach

For this approach, a beech-chair position is elected verifying head elevation of 30° and under general anesthesia. Head must be properly secured, and the arm placed on a lateral arm table/board for support. Preoperative intravenous antibiotic prophylaxis should be dispensed 30 min before the incision. C-arm fluoroscope images are obtained to ensure appropriate radiologic shoulder views (true AP, axillary and scapular Y views). The arm is cleaned and draped in a sterile fashion making sure the hand and forearm are appropriately insulated. Suitable skin exposure of the shoulder and axilla must be confirmed. Incision is marked, and local anesthetic with epinephrine is recommended to limit bleeding during surgical dissection. A vertical incision is made from the inferior border of the coracoid process and carried down to the axillary skin fold (~8 cm approximately). The deltopectoral intermuscular plane is recognized and split, the pectoralis major muscle is retracted medially, while the deltoid muscle belly and cephalic vein are retracted laterally. To access the anterior border of the GH joint, the conjoint tendon is recognized and retracted medially. If necessary, an osteotomy of the coracoid process tip can be performed to facilitate the medial retraction of the conjoint tendon. Following, the arm should be in external rotation, as this will open a window to visualize the subscapularis tendon, which is repaired with stay sutures before the tenotomy. Before deep capsulotomy, caution and appropriate ligation of humeral circumflex arteries at the inferior border must be ensured. Subscapularis tenodesis is then made within 1–2 cm proximal to the insertion at the lesser humeral tubercle. Capsulotomy is completed on a vertical fashion, following the medial aspect of the subscapularis stump. For appropriate glenoid exposure, two Hohmman retractors are placed on the superior and inferior glenoid neck, and a third retractor (Fukuda) mobilizing the humeral head laterally should allow suitable exposure of the anterior aspect of the glenoid fossa. Once the fracture is recognized, cleaned and appropriate reduction is attained, temporary fixation with small diameter K-wires is recommended. Before definitive fixation with either cannulated headless, cortical screws, or minifragment plates, confirmation under fluoroscopy will verify proper reduction and extra-articular screw placement. Labral tears can reconstruct in place with anchors and/or resistant non-absorbable sutures. Irrigation and hemostasis must be completed before closure. The capsule and subscapularis tendon can be closed in a continuous manner with a running suture. Subcutaneous and skin closure can be finished with interrupted sutures [21] (Fig. 7.7).

Figure 7.8 shows the reduction and provisional fixation of a glenoid fracture using the axillary approach.

Figures 7.9 and 7.10 illustrate the treatment of glenoid rim fractures using the axillary approach.

Certain glenoid fracture configurations are managed using posterior approaches. Depending on the fracture pattern, the extension into the scapular neck or body, and degree of displacement, one can consider using the Brodsky, classic or modified

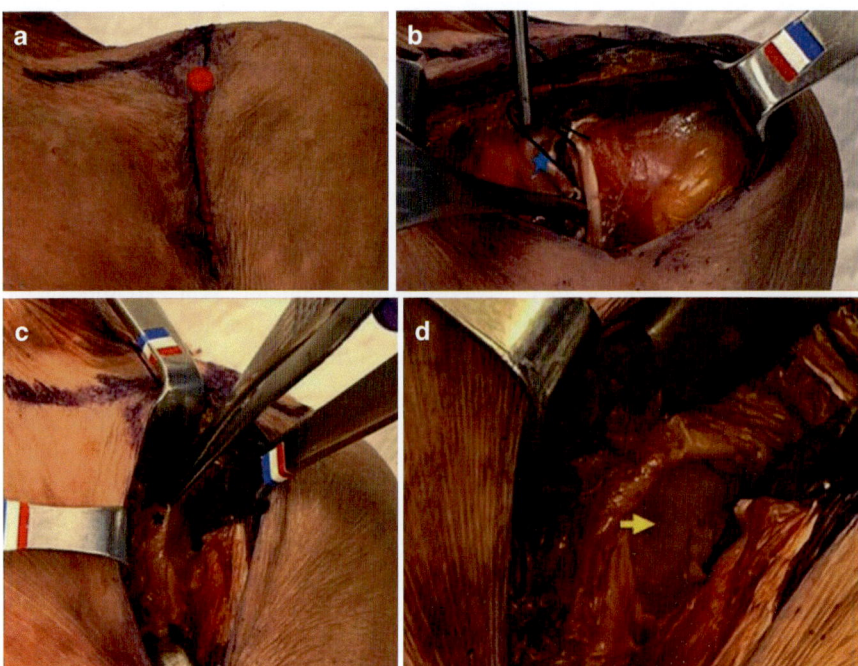

Fig. 7.7 Cadaveric dissection showing the steps of the vertical anterior axillary incision described by Leslie and Ryan [22]. (**a**) Skin incision begins inferior to the tip of the coracoid (red circle) and progresses toward the anterior axillary fold. (**b**) The deltopectoral interval is identified, and the superficial muscle structures and the cephalic vein are retracted, as well as the conjoint tendon. The subscapularis tendon is tagged with stay sutures. (**c**) The joint is exposed after the subscapularis tenotomy and the incision of the capsule. The asterisk depicts the anterior labrum. (**d**) Hohmann retractors are positioned superiorly and inferiorly to the glenoid surface, and a Fukuda or Hohmann retractor lateralizes the humeral head, exposing the anterior half of the glenoid fossa

Judet, or posteriorly oriented minimally invasive approaches to achieve adequate fracture reduction and fixation [21, 23]. In our practice, we consider the use a posterior approach for fractures within the posterior rim fractures carrying >25% of the glenoid fossa and for all other posteriorly oriented glenoid fossa fracture patterns. Currently, combined limited or minimally invasive approaches are desirable [23, 24]. When associated, the medial pillar component of the scapular fracture should be reduced and fixed with a relatively flexible implant first as it acts as a hinge to allow better manipulation, reduction, and final fixation of the lateral pillar component. Conventional or locked 3.5-mm small fragment plates and screws, as well as minifragment plates and screws (2.0, 2.4, or 2.7 mm) can be used for fracture fixation. A long 3.5-mm cortical screw can be placed in a posterior-to-anterior direction to fix the base of the coracoid process, if necessary.

7 Special Considerations: Articular Involvement (Glenoid Fossa and Rim) 67

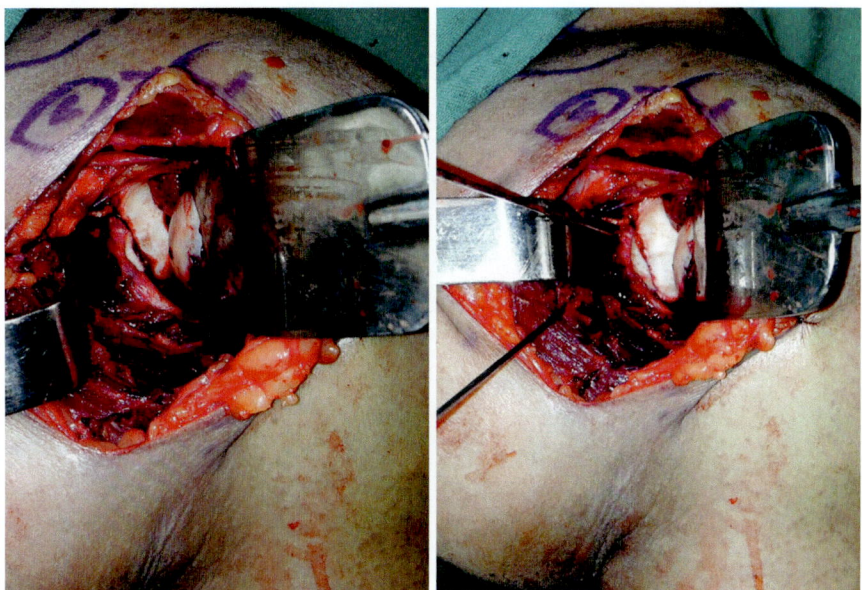

Fig. 7.8 Intraoperative photographs demonstrating the reduction and provisional fixation of a glenoid fracture using the axillary approach

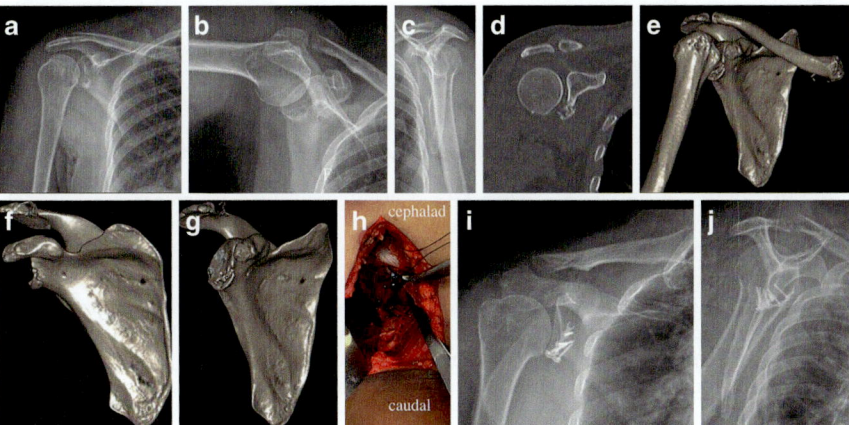

Fig. 7.9 A 68-year-old female patient presented the first incident of shoulder dislocation. After joint reduction, the shoulder remained unstable. (**a–c**): Radiographs of the right shoulder in anteroposterior, axillary, and Y views showing reduction of the dislocation. (**d**): CT scan in coronal cut showing the glenoid fracture (Ideberg 1a). (**e–g**): 3D CT scan showing the Ideberg 1a fracture pattern. (**h**): Intraoperative photograph showing the rim plate placement for fracture fixation. Radiographs in anteroposterior (**i**) and Y (**j**) views showing fracture reduction and fixation with the 2.0-mm rim plate

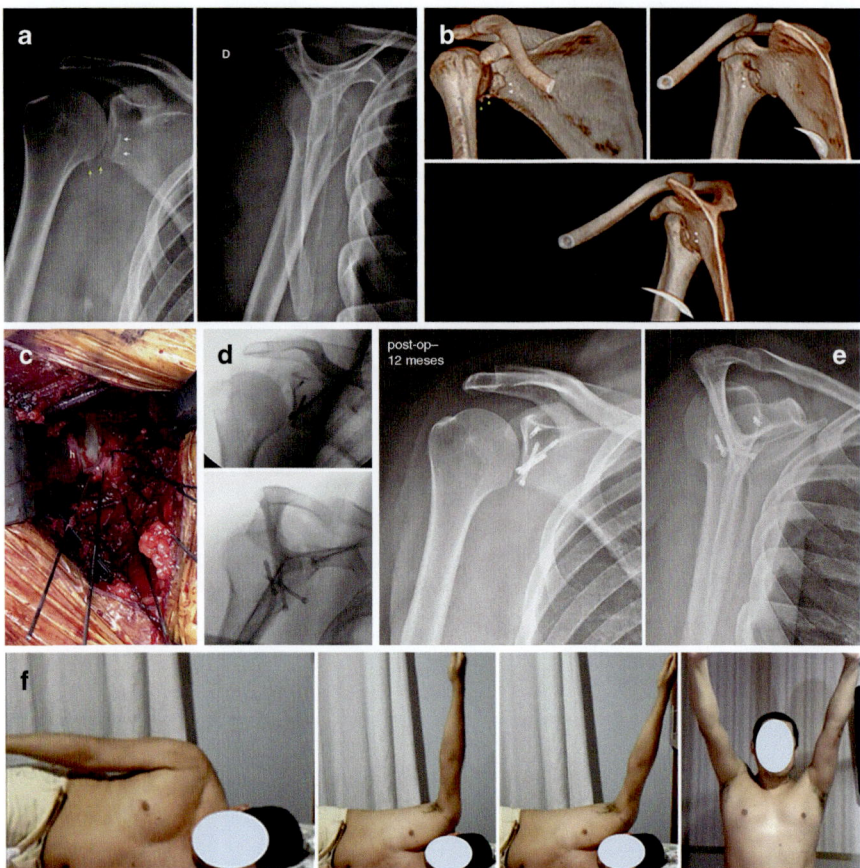

Fig. 7.10 (**a**): Preoperative images in true AP and lateral scapular radiographic views of the right shoulder of a 40-years-old male patient, showing a step-off on the anteroinferior rim of the glenoid. (**b**): Preoperative 3-D CT reconstructions showing the displaced anteroinferior glenoid rim fracture and small bone fragments in the inferior portion of the capsule; (**c**): Intraoperative image showing the anteroinferior rim fracture anatomically reduced and provisionally fixed with multiple threaded K-wires. Observe the number 2 ethibond® sutures attached to the anterior labrum for posterior repair. *—anteroinferior glenoid rim fragment, h—humerus head; (**d**): Intraoperative true AP and lateral scapular fluoroscopic views of the right shoulder showing final fixation with three 2.4-mm headless screws. Labrum was repaired using a bone anchor and unabsorbable sutures; (**e**): Postoperative true anteroposterior and lateral scapular radiographic views of the right shoulder demonstrating the anatomic reduction of the anterior glenoid rim; (**f**): Pictures done during the rehabilitation protocol, demonstrating a satisfactory range of motion of the operated shoulder

For Ideberg type 3 glenoid fractures, we usually address the fracture percutaneously or using a mini-open skin incision, use a K-wire through the coracoid process to manipulate and reduce the fracture and insert a long cortical or cannulated 3.5 mm screw from anterior-cephalad to posterior-caudal direction (Fig. 7.11).

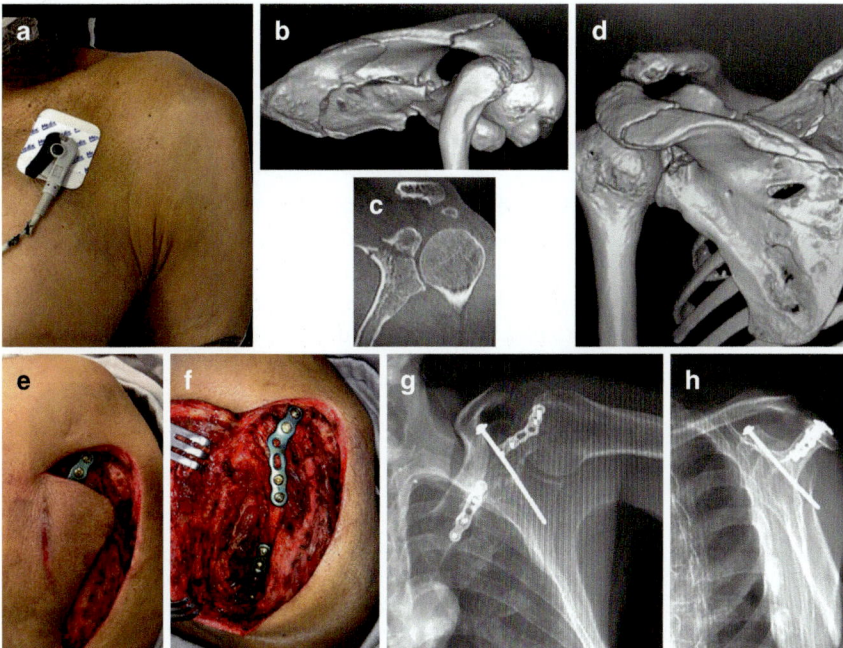

Fig. 7.11 (**a**): Observe the clinical aspect of the deformity on the left shoulder of the patient after a motorcycle accident. (**b–d**): CT scan showing the associated glenoid, acromion, and scapular spine fracture. (**e** and **f**): A superior "L-shaped" approach developed to address all fractures. Observe the fixation of the acromion and the scapular spine fractures with 2.4-mm minifragment plates. (**g** and **h**): Radiographs showing fracture reduction and fixation. Observe the placement of the screw into the coracoid process and glenoid corridor

7.7 Rehabilitation Protocol

Once appropriate stable fixation is confirmed with radiographs and or CT scans, a two-phase rehabilitation protocol can be initiated. Phase 1 should start as early as postoperative day 1 with active and assisted ROM exercises as tolerated, this phase will continue up to 10 weeks. These exercises can be performed either sitting or in a supine position in bed. If the axillary approach was performed, emphasis on the importance of restricting shoulder external rotation movements during this early stage must comprehended to avoid excessive forces at the repair site. Involvement and collaboration with the inpatient physical therapy team are mandatory to ensure proper rehabilitation techniques before hospital discharge. Phase 2 usually starts around 10 weeks after surgery once the labrum and fracture have healed. Rehabilitation goals during phase 2 include proprioception, strengthening, and ROM exercises with added elastic resistance or weight as tolerated. If a posterior approach was performed and the fracture fixation is considered stable, both passive and active exercises are stimulated to regain progressive range of motion and proprioception of the operated shoulder as soon as adequate pain control is achieved. Also, patients are advised to exercise the ipsilateral elbow, wrist, and fingers and to avoid heavy objects with the operated upper limb during a minimum of 6 weeks after the surgical procedure. Progressive strengthening is started after this period until bone healing.

On average, five postoperative clinic visits are recommended within the first year, set at 3, 6, and 12 weeks, and then followed every 6 months during first year. Plain radiographs are recommended on every visit to assess fracture healing and rule out any ongoing complications. Finally, functional outcome evaluation is encouraged in all patients to objectively measure improvement, functionality, and achievement of postoperative goals [21].

References

1. Seidl AJ, Joyce CD. Acute fractures of the glenoid. J Am Acad Orthop Surg. 2020;28(22):e978–87. https://doi.org/10.5435/JAAOS-D-20-00252. PMID: 33156084.
2. Frich LH, Larsen MS. How to deal with a glenoid fracture. EFORT Open Rev. 2017;2(5):151–7. https://doi.org/10.1302/2058-5241.2.160082.
3. Königshausen M, Coulibaly MO, Nicolas V, Schildhauer TA, Seybold D. Results of non-operative treatment of fractures of the glenoid fossa. Bone Joint J. 2016;98-B(8):1074–9. https://doi.org/10.1302/0301-620X.98B8.35687. PMID: 27482020.
4. Goss TP. Fractures of the glenoid cavity. J Bone Joint Surg Am. 1992;74(2):299–305. PMID: 1541626.
5. Bragg KJ, Tapscott DC, Varacallo M. Glenoid fractures. In: StatPearls [Internet]. Treasure Island: StatPearls; 2023. PMID: 31335046.
6. Piponov HI, Savin D, Shah N, Esposito D, Schwartz B, Moretti V, Goldberg B. Glenoid version and size: does gender, ethnicity, or body size play a role? Int Orthop. 2016;40(11):2347–53. https://doi.org/10.1007/s00264-016-3201-8. Epub 2016 Apr 22. PMID: 27106214.
7. Matsumura N, Ogawa K, Kobayashi S, Oki S, Watanabe A, Ikegami H, Toyama Y. Morphologic features of humeral head and glenoid version in the normal glenohumeral joint. J Shoulder Elb Surg. 2014;23(11):1724–30. https://doi.org/10.1016/j.jse.2014.02.020. Epub 2014 May 24. PMID: 24862249.
8. Abrassart S, Stern R, Hoffmeyer P. Arterial supply of the glenoid: an anatomic study. J Shoulder Elb Surg. 2006;15(2):232–8. https://doi.org/10.1016/j.jse.2005.07.015.
9. Lantry JM, Roberts CS, Giannoudis PV. Operative treatment of scapular fractures: a systematic review. Injury. 2008;39(3):271–83. https://doi.org/10.1016/j.injury.2007.06.018. Epub 2007 Oct 4. PMID: 17919636.
10. ter Meulen DP, Janssen SJ, Hageman MG, Ring DC. Quantitative three-dimensional computed tomography analysis of glenoid fracture patterns according to the AO/OTA classification. J Shoulder Elb Surg. 2016;25(2):269–75. https://doi.org/10.1016/j.jse.2015.07.022. Epub 2015 Oct 9. PMID: 26456425.
11. Harris RD, Harris JH Jr. The prevalence and significance of missed scapular fractures in blunt chest trauma. AJR Am J Roentgenol. 1988;151(4):747–50. https://doi.org/10.2214/ajr.151.4.747. PMID: 3262275.
12. Kelly MJ, Holton AE, Cassar-Gheiti AJ, Hanna SA, Quinlan JF, Molony DC. The aetiology of posterior glenohumeral dislocations and occurrence of associated injuries: a systematic review. Bone Joint J. 2019;101-B(1):15–21. https://doi.org/10.1302/0301-620X.101B1.BJJ-2018-0984.R1. PMID: 30601057.

13. Thakkar RS, Thakkar SC, Srikumaran U, McFarland EG, Fayad LM. Complications of rotator cuff surgery-the role of post-operative imaging in patient care. Br J Radiol. 2014;87(1039):20130630. https://doi.org/10.1259/bjr.20130630. Epub 2014 Apr 15. PMID: 24734935; PMCID: PMC4075575
14. Gilbert F, Eden L, Meffert R, Konietschke F, Lotz J, Bauer L, Staab W. Intra- and interobserver reliability of glenoid fracture classifications by Ideberg, Euler and AO. BMC Musculoskelet Disord. 2018;19(1):89. https://doi.org/10.1186/s12891-018-2016-8. PMID: 29580228; PMCID: PMC5870213.
15. Ideberg R, Grevsten S, Larsson S. Epidemiology of scapular fractures. Incidence and classification of 338 fractures. Acta Orthop Scand. 1995;66(5):395–7. https://doi.org/10.3109/17453679508995571. PMID: 7484114.
16. Jaeger M, Lambert S, Südkamp NP, Kellam JF, Madsen JE, Babst R, Andermahr J, Li W, Audigé L. The AO Foundation and Orthopaedic Trauma Association (AO/OTA) scapula fracture classification system: focus on glenoid fossa involvement. J Shoulder Elb Surg. 2013;22(4):512–20. https://doi.org/10.1016/j.jse.2012.08.003. Epub 2012 Sep 28. PMID: 23021902.
17. Harvey E, Audigé L, Herscovici D Jr, Agel J, Madsen JE, Babst R, Nork S, Kellam J. Development and validation of the new international classification for scapula fractures. J Orthop Trauma. 2012;26(6):364–9. https://doi.org/10.1097/BOT.0b013e3182382625. PMID: 22430519.
18. Bartoníček J, Tuček M, Klika D, Chochola A. Pathoanatomy and computed tomography classification of glenoid fossa fractures based on ninety patients. Int Orthop. 2016;40:2383–92. https://doi.org/10.1007/s00264-016-3169-4.
19. Mayo KA, Benirschke SK, Mast JW. Displaced fractures of the glenoid fossa. Results of open reduction and internal fixation. Clin Orthop Relat Res. 1998;(347):122–30. PMID: 9520882.
20. Cole PA, Gauger EM, Herrera DA, Anavian J, Tarkin IS. Radiographic follow-up of 84 operatively treated scapula neck and body fractures. Injury. 2012;43(3):327–33. https://doi.org/10.1016/j.injury.2011.09.029. Epub 2011 Oct 27. PMID: 22036452.
21. Giordano V, Pires RE, Labronici PJ, Vieira I, de Souza FS, Sassine TJ, et al. Open reduction and internal fixation of Ideberg type IA glenoid fractures: tricks, pearls, and potential pitfalls based on a retrospective cohort of 33 patients focusing on the rehabilitation protocol. Eur J Orthop Surg Traumatol. 2023;33(3):571–80. https://doi.org/10.1007/s00590-022-03389-7. Epub 2022 Sep 12. PMID: 36094673.
22. Leslie JT Jr, Ryan TJ. The anterior axillary incision to approach the shoulder joint. J Bone Joint Surg. 1962;44(6):1193–6.
23. Pires RE, Giordano V, de Souza FSM, Labronici PJ. Current challenges and controversies in the management of scapular fractures: a review. Patient Saf Surg. 2021;15(1):6. https://doi.org/10.1186/s13037-020-00281-3. PMID: 33407725; PMCID: PMC7789406.
24. Gauger EM, Cole PA. Surgical technique: a minimally invasive approach to scapula neck and body fractures. Clin Orthop Relat Res. 2011;469(12):3390–9. https://doi.org/10.1007/s11999-011-1970-3. PMID: 21761253; PMCID: PMC3210267.

Chapter 8
Special Considerations: Fractures of the Coracoid Process and Acromion

Pedro José Labronici, Robinson Esteves Pires, and Vincenzo Giordano

8.1 Coracoid Process Fractures

The coracoid process presents three main functions: it serves as a point of muscles and tendons attachment; contributes to the anterior superior stability of the glenohumeral joint; and is part of the superior shoulder suspensory complex (SSSC) [1–3]. The coracoid process fracture is a rare injury. McGinnis and Denton [4] described the prevalence of coracoid fractures between 3% and 13% of all scapular fractures. More recent data from two systematic reviews of scapular fractures reported the prevalence of apophyseal acromion and coracoid process fractures at 6% and 8.2%, respectively [5, 6]. Fractures of the coracoid process are typically caused by high-energy trauma, generally associated with other fractures and/or disruption of the SSSC, especially the acromioclavicular joint [7–10] (Fig. 8.1).

8.1.1 Anatomy

From the scapular origin, the coracoid process projects cranially and anterolaterally, but then turns with the tip projecting anteriorly and inferiorly, with a curved undersurface. Along the superior portion, from medial to lateral, the attachments are the

---

P. J. Labronici
Department of General and Specialized Surgery, Fluminense Federal University, Niterói, Brazil

R. E. Pires (✉)
Department of the Locomotor Apparatus, Federal University of Minas Gerais, Belo Horizonte, Minas Gerais, Brazil

V. Giordano
Orthopedics Department, Hospital Municipal Miguel Couto, Rio de Janeiro, Brazil

© The Author(s), under exclusive license to Springer Nature Switzerland AG 2024
R. E. Pires et al. (eds.), *Fractures of the Scapula*,
https://doi.org/10.1007/978-3-031-58498-5_8

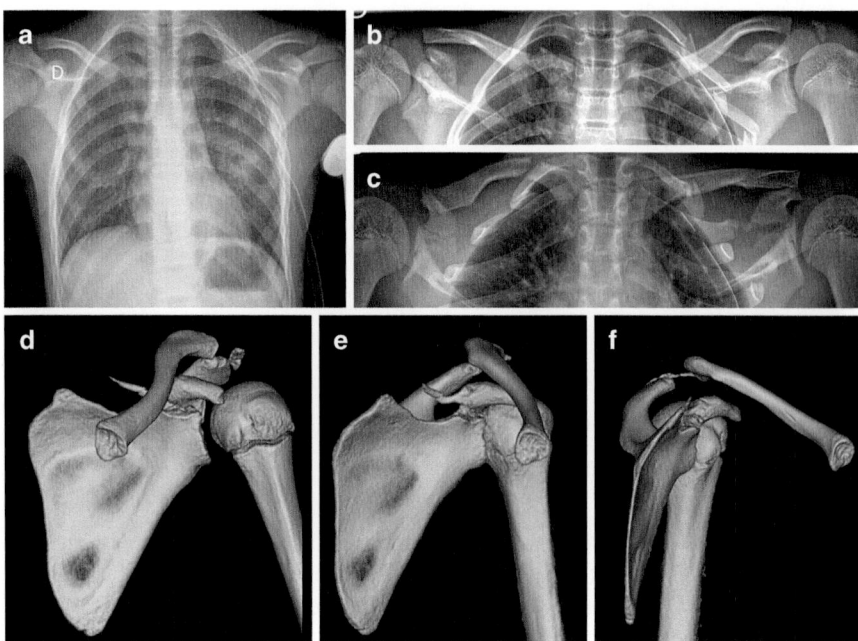

Fig. 8.1 Radiographs of the chest (**a**) and acromioclavicular joints (**b** and **c**) showing the rib fractures, medial-third clavicle fracture (right shoulder), and coracoid base fracture with associated acromioclavicular dislocation (left shoulder). CT scan with 3D reconstruction details the coracoid base fracture with associated acromioclavicular dislocation (**d–f**)

transverse scapular ligament, coracoclavicular ligaments, and the coracoacromial ligament. The coracoacromial ligament is responsible, along with the pectoralis minor, for preventing the coracoid process from displacing inferiorly. The coracoid process develops as a primary ossification center in the first year of life, progressively enlarges, and fuses with the scapula around the age of 14–15 years [11, 12]. A separate physis forms at the tip of the coracoid and permits longitudinal growth, closing between ages 18 and 25 years. These physis should not be mistaken with fractures. In patients under 25 years of age, the disruption to the coracoid physis may lead to a nonunion scenario [12].

8.1.2 Injury Mechanism

Fractures of the coracoid process generally occur due to three different trauma mechanisms. The first due to direct high-energy trauma caused by a vehicular accident or falls over the shoulder [7, 9, 13, 14]. The most common associated injuries are acromioclavicular dislocation, glenohumeral injury, rotator cuff injury, acromion fracture, distal third of the clavicle fracture, scapular fracture, and humeral fractures [7, 9]. This mechanism results in a combination of lesions proposed by Wilson and Colwill [15], which involves direct forces on the acromioclavicular joint, causing a caudal displacement of the acromion and scapula, whereas the coracoclavicular ligaments pull the coracoid process in a cephalad direction. Coracoid process fracture may be caused by an abrupt contraction of the conjoint tendon and pectoralis minor muscle, and residual forces on the coracoclavicular ligament may determine its disruption. A second mechanism, more rare, is caused by avulsion of the coracoid process due to a sudden eccentric contraction of the muscles attached on the coracoid process (short head of the biceps, coracobrachialis, and pectoralis minor muscles) and by the coracoclavicular ligaments [11, 15–19]. A third mechanism, also extremely rare, is the fatigue fracture of the coracoid process, usually caused by repetitive microtrauma, mainly in athletes [20].

8.1.3 Classification

Several classification systems were proposed for coracoid process fractures. In the Ogawa [7] classification system, the type I fracture is proximal to the coracoclavicular ligament attachment, while the type II fracture is distal. Eyres and Brooks [9] proposed a more detailed classification system, based on a review of 12 coracoid process fractures. In the classification by Eyres, coracoid fractures are divided into five types and subgrouped into A or B, according to the presence or absence of associated injuries to the clavicle or its ligamentous connection that affects scapular stability. On Type I, the coracoid fracture involves the tip or epiphyseal area. Type II is midprocess fracture. Type III is a fracture of the basis of the coracoid process. On Type IV, the superior body of the scapula is involved. On Type V, fracture extends into the glenoid fossa. Bartoníček et al. [21] developed a classification based on 3D-CT reconstructions. Type I is a fracture of apex; Type II is a fracture of beak; Type III is a fracture of basis; Type IV is a comminuted pattern.

8.1.4 Treatment

8.1.4.1 Nonoperative Treatment

Isolated, nondisplaced, or minimally displaced coracoid process fractures can be successfully treated with nonoperative management [22–24]. Even with displacement, isolated coracoid tip fractures (Eyres type 1) and fracture between the coracoclavicular and coracoacromial ligaments (Eyres type 2 to 3) can be successfully treated with nonsurgical management [7, 9, 10].

8.1.4.2 Operative Treatment

Indications for operative management may include symptomatic nonunion, more than 1 cm displacement, and multiple disruption of the SSSC [25, 26]. In prior studies, most operative indications were secondary to injuries of the SSSC [7, 25]. It is important to recognize the combination of an injury to the coracoid process with another injury to the SSSC, since it represents a double disruption of the SSSC, which creates an unstable anatomical situation that can result in persistent functional disability of the shoulder [2, 25, 26]. Additionally, in fractures that are distal to the coracoclavicular ligament, the distal fracture fragment can be inferiorly displaced by the force of the conjoint tendon and ligaments. Figure 8.2 depicts a coracoid process fracture, which extends toward the body of the scapula and glenoid. This fracture pattern is generally unstable and presents an important shear mechanism due to impingement of the humeral head or clavicle. Furthermore, there is a risk of compression on the plexus, which can affect both the nervous and arterial structures [27].

The first concern on the preoperative planning is the positioning of the C-arm. It should preferably be positioned on the opposite side of the table, in order to get orthogonal images. By positioning the patient on a radiolucent table, it allows the surgeon to obtain a good quality scapular-Y and Stryker notch fluoroscopic views, which are extremely helpful to verify fracture reduction and correct screw placement. Several approaches were described for the treatment of coracoid process fractures, including the standard deltopectoral, infraclavicular, and transclavicular

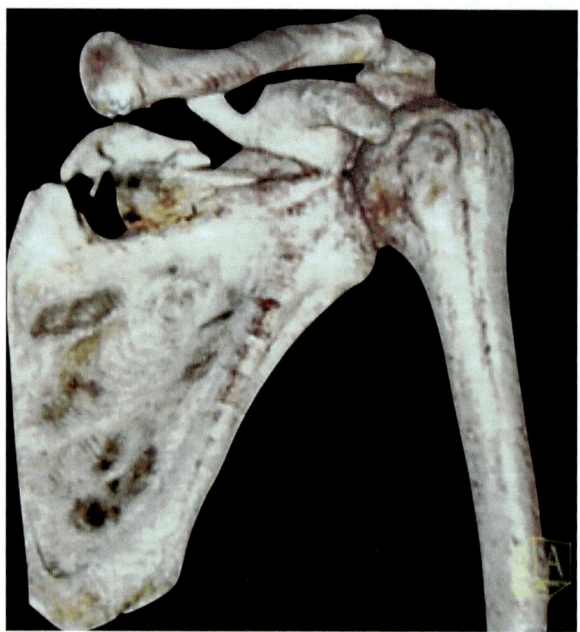

Fig. 8.2 3D CT scan showing the coracoid process inferiorly displaced by the short head of the biceps, coracobrachialis, and pectoralis minor muscles

8 Special Considerations: Fractures of the Coracoid Process and Acromion

(when a clavicle fracture at the level of the coracoid process is associated) approaches [28–30]. Using the standard deltopectoral approach, open reduction of the coracoid process fracture, we must consider a screw correctly placed down into the coracoid tunnel [28, 30]. Some critical points deserve to be highlighted:

1. To correct the anterior and medial rotatory displacement of the coracoid, a suture is carefully positioned at the origin of the conjoint tendon. An assistant then pulls this suture in the craniomedial direction while ensuring that the patient's elbow remains flexed. Subsequently, temporarily fixate with a K-wire, assess reduction via fluoroscopy, and perform final fixation with a screw [31] (Figs. 8.3 and 8.4).
2. The screw must be placed down the coracoid stalk, through the coracoid base and into the neck of the scapula. In most cases, the drill must be positioned perpendicular to the coracoid process and parallel to the longest axis of the glenoid cavity. To prevent a drill bit breakage, one can alternatively use a 2.5 mm K-wire. This k-wire can be used as a joystick to manipulate the coracoid process, to achieve adequate reduction.
3. The screw must be placed parallel to the glenoid fossa.
4. The screw must be placed without violating or penetrating the bony borders of the coracoid tunnel. The 3.5 mm cortical screw (as a lag screw or positioning screw if comminution is present) or the 3.5 mm cannulated screw can be used to fix the coracoid process fracture (Fig. 8.5). Figure 8.6 illustrates the treatment of an associated coracoid process and clavicle fracture.

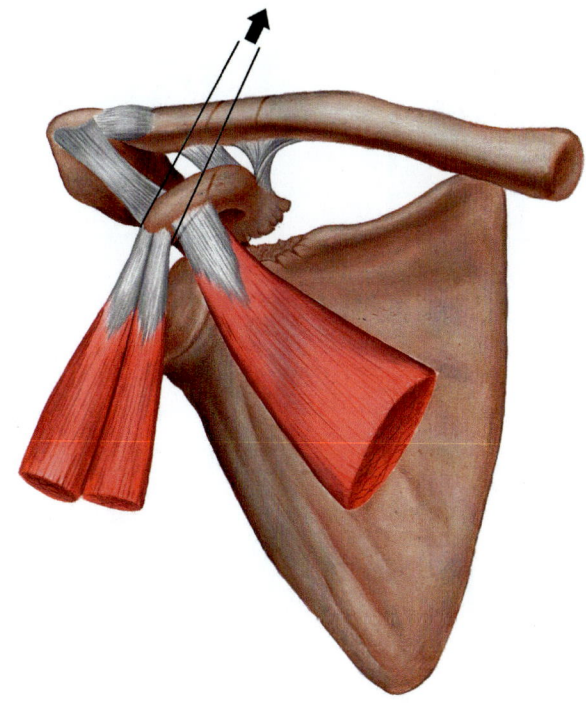

Fig. 8.3 Correction the rotatory displacement of the coracoid with suture (arrow) positioned at the origin of the conjoint tendon. An assistant pulls this suture in the craniomedial direction

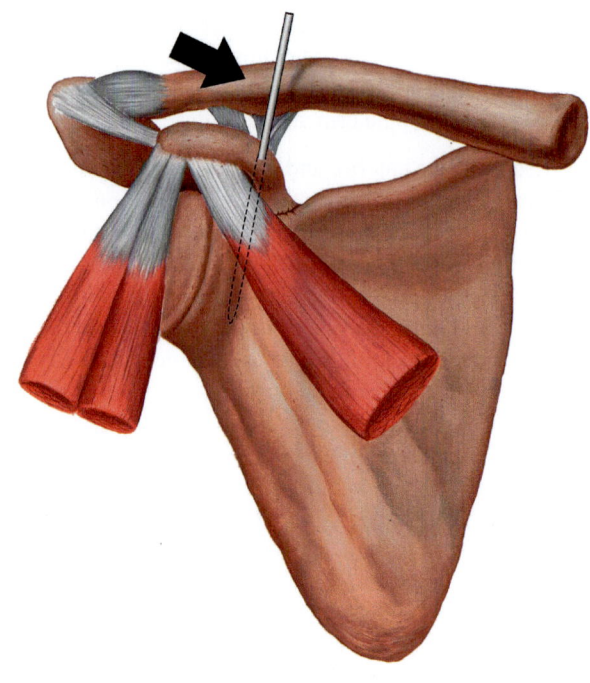

Fig. 8.4 Temporary fracture fixation with a K-wire (arrow). It is recommended to assess reduction using fluoroscopic images (Y and Stryker views)

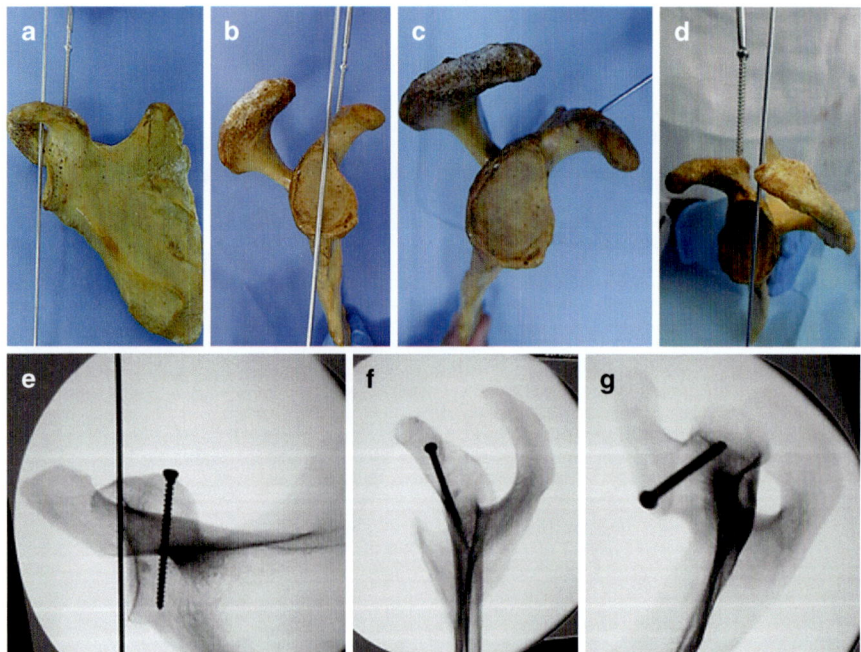

Fig. 8.5 Observe the correct placement of the screw into the corridor of the coracoid process (**a–d**). Fluoroscopy images confirm the correct pathway of the screw (**e–g**)

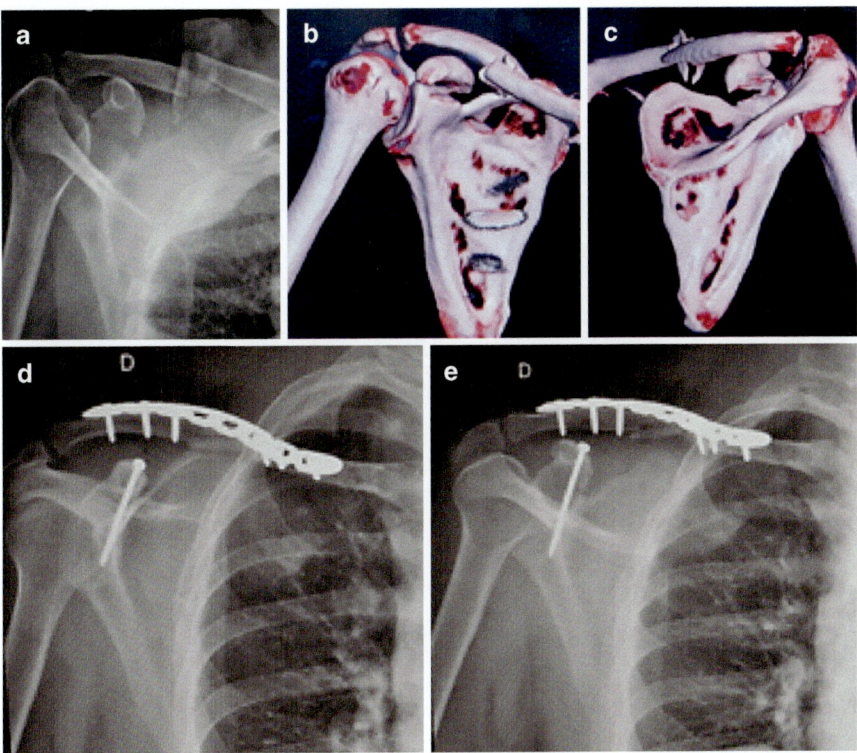

Fig. 8.6 (a) Radiograph of the right shoulder in anteroposterior view with cephalad inclination showing the associated fracture of the coracoid process and clavicle. (b and c) 3D CT scan showing the combined fracture. (d and e) Postoperative radiographs showing the fixation of the coracoid process with a 3.5 mm cortical screw and the clavicle fixation with a 3.5 precontoured LCP plate

Figure 8.7 illustrates the treatment of a patient who suffered a vehicle accident and presented a combined coracoid process, acromion, and scapular spine fracture. Figure 8.8 illustrates a complex fracture of the scapula (coracoid process, scapular spine, and body). Observe the displacement of the coracoid process and the bifocal fracture pattern of this bone (avulsion fracture of the coracoid tip associated with the coracoid basis).

Ogawa et al. [7] retrospectively reviewed 67 patients with isolated coracoid fractures. Forty-five patients were available for a follow-up at a mean of 37 months (12–117 months). No notable difference was observed in the outcomes between patients with type 1 and 2 fractures and between those undergoing nonoperative or operative treatment. Hill et al. [28] analyzed the outcomes of 22 patients with isolated coracoid process fractures treated operatively. A total of 17 patients underwent open reduction and fixation with 1–3 lag screws, whereas 5 patients underwent surgical fixation with a combination of screws and a small plate. At a mean follow-up of 23.5 months, the median Disabilities of the Arm, Shoulder, and Hand (DASH)

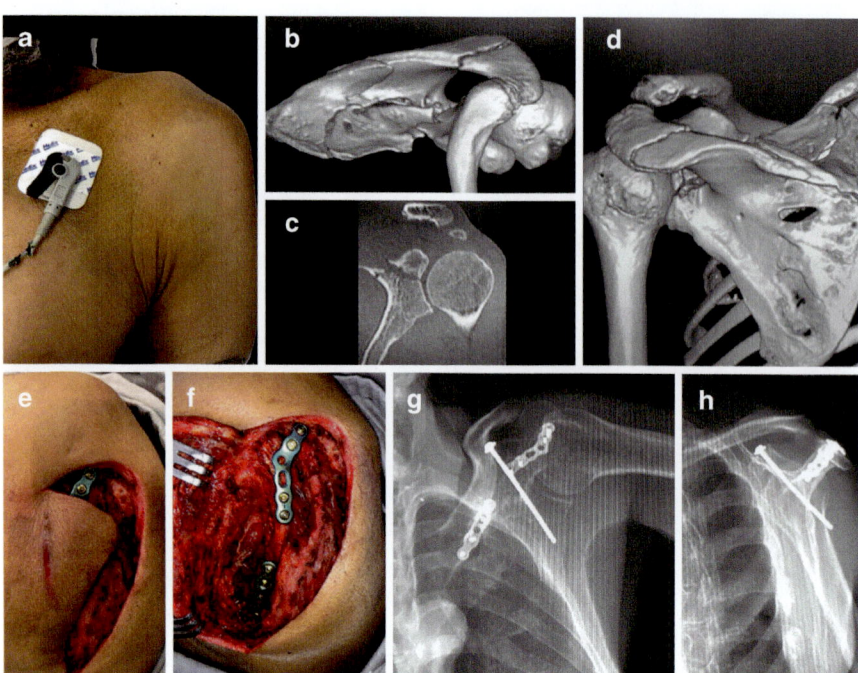

Fig. 8.7 (**a**) Observe the clinical aspect of the deformity on the left shoulder of the patient. (**b–d**) CT scan showing the associated coracoid process, acromion, and scapular spine fracture. (**e** and **f**) Superior "L-shaped" developed to address all fractures. Observe the fixation of the acromion and the scapular spine with 2.4 minifragment plates. (**g** and **h**) Radiographs showing fixation of the fractures. Observe the placement of the screw into the coracoid process corridor

score was 12.3 (range: 0–74; mean = 10.1) and 16 (84%). According to Galvin et al. [27], surgical fixation is indicated if coracoid fractures are associated with an unstable SSSC, displaced extension into either the scapula body or glenoid fossa, or progression into a painful nonunion. However, the decision between nonoperative management versus operative intervention should be a shared decision between the patient and the surgeon, based on the fracture pattern, associated shoulder injuries, patient's activity or sporting level, and future expectations.

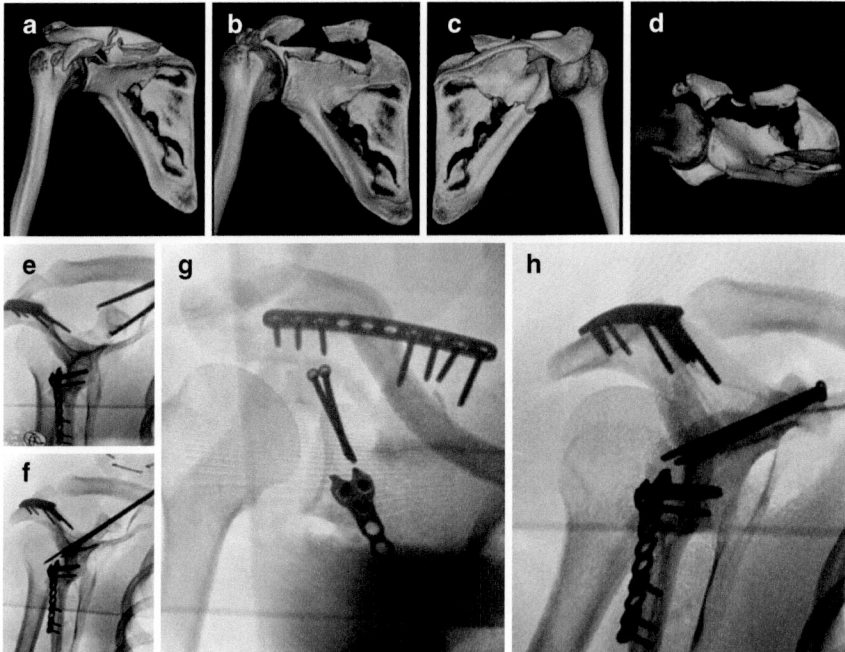

Fig. 8.8 (**a–d**) 3D CT scan demonstrating a complex scapular fracture. Observe the bifocal pattern of the coracoid process and the association with the scapular spine and body fractures. Fixation was performed initially with the patient prone, using 2 minimally invasive approaches to address the scapular spine and the lateral pillar of the scapula. Afterwards, the patient was placed supine, and an anterior approach (deltopectoral) was used to reduce (**e** and **f**) and fix the coracoid process fracture with two 2.7 mm lag screws (**g** and **h**). A transosseous suture was performed to reattach the tip of the coracoid process and the conjoint tendon

8.2 Acromion Fractures

Acromion are rare and affect approximately 8–16% of all scapular fractures [30, 32, 33]. The injury mescanism can be an indirect trauma, caused by the muscles attached into the acromion or a direct high-energy trauma, over the lateral surface of the shoulder. These fractures are frequently associated with fractures of the ipsilateral glenoid, neck, and body of the scapula, clavicle, rib with or without lung injury, spine fracture, brachial plexus injury, humeral fracture, and cerebral contusion [34–38] (Fig. 8.9).

Fractures of the acromion represent a challenge for diagnosis and treatment [30, 39, 40]. As acromion fractures are usually associated with other shoulder and thoracic injuries, a delay in diagnosis may be present. Furthermore, these fractures may not be identified on conventional radiographs or may be confused with os acromiale, which is present in approximately 3% of the population [30, 39].

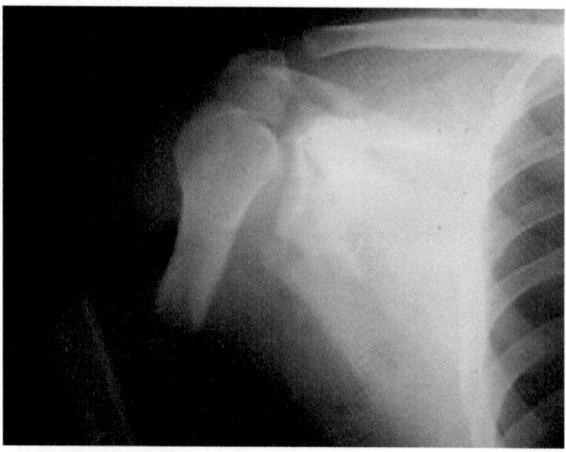

Fig. 8.9 Radiograph of the right shoulder in anteroposterior view showing a displaced fracture of the acromion, in combination to a scapular neck fracture and a diaphyseal fracture of the humerus due to high-energy trauma

Two classification systems are universally used for acromion fractures. Ogawa and Naniwa [40] proposed a simple and anatomical classification. Type I represents a fracture in the lateral region of the acromion. Type II represents a fracture medial to the acromion with a descending line toward the spinoglenoid notch. Kuhn et al. [41], in a case series of 27 acromion fractures managed nonoperatively, classified acromion fractures into three types. Type I is a minimally displaced acromion fracture. Type II is a laterally displaced fracture. Type III is a displaced fracture of the acromion with reduction of the subacromial space.

8.2.1 Treatment

Unfortunately, there is no consensus to guide the treatment of acromion fractures.

8.2.1.1 Nonoperative Management

The acromion is a structure with multiple ligament and muscle attachments. The coracoacromial ligament extends from the basis of the coracoid process anteriorly to the inferior surface of the acromion, within the subacromial space. The trapezius muscle attaches distally in the acromion and has the function of retracting the scapula and rotating the glenoid cavity superiorly. The deltoid muscle attaches proximally to the acromion and works mainly to abduct the arm. Therefore, nonoperative treatment should be indicated for stable and nondisplaced fractures. However, the patient should be closed monitored due to the risk of secondary displacement. Complications associated with the nonoperative management of displaced acromion fractures include pain, decreased motion, rotator cuff tears secondary to subacromial impingement, acromioclavicular joint dislocation, humeral head subluxation, shoulder weakness, brachial plexus injury, and symptomatic nonunion [30]. Gorczyca et al. [37] reported that although nonoperative treatment of displaced acromion fractures generally results in satisfactory shoulder function, no studies have measured shoulder strength after nonoperative treatment of displaced fractures of the acromion.

8.2.1.2 Operative Management

Indications for the operative treatment of acromion fractures are controversial in the current literature [30, 31–34]. A review of the surgical treatment of acromion fractures revealed a variety of fixation techniques, including fixation with K-wires, tension band wiring, fixation with screws, fixation with plates, and arthroscopically assisted fixation [30, 32–40]. Hardegger et al. [32] recommended osteosynthesis of acromion fractures in fractures with significant displacement to prevent painful nonunion and protect the rotator cuff from impact. Ringelberg [42] demonstrated that the mean force generated by the middle third of the deltoid keeping the arm at 45 degrees of abduction is greater than 400 Newtons. Therefore, there is considerable traction of the deltoid muscle on the acromion, even with unresisted shoulder movement. Bauer et al. [34] and McGahan and Rab [36] recommended fixation for fractures of the acromion with marked displacement, after considering the patient's age, activity, and clinical status.

Based on the classification scheme proposed by Kuhn et al. [41], operative treatment should be considered for patients with Type III fractures and symptomatic nonunions in Type II fractures. Figure 8.10 illustrates the treatment of a type III acromion. Bauer et al. [34] proposed that, particularly in fractures with compromised subacromial space, anatomic restoration may prevent muscular dysfunction

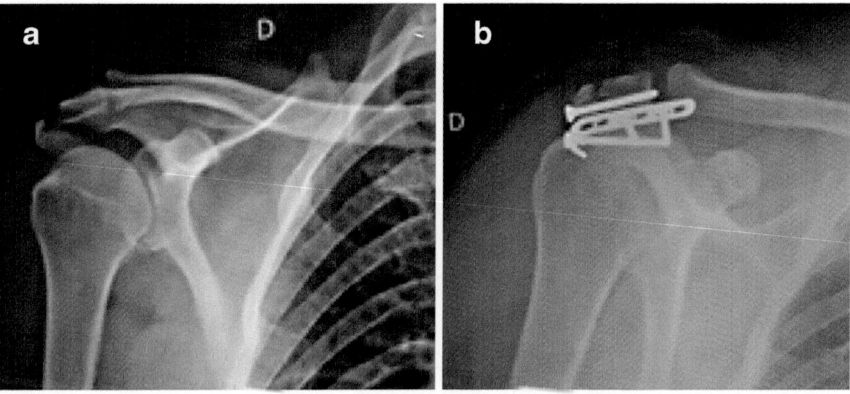

Fig. 8.10 (**a**) Radiograph of the right shoulder showing a Type III fracture, according to the Kuhn classification system. Observe the subacromial space. (**b**) Fracture reduction and fixation with minifragment plate and screws

and scapular dyskinesia. Kim et al. [43] compared early and delayed fixation in a retrospective series of 34 patients and found a significantly better constant score and daily activity score in the early fixation group. Hess et al. [44] developed a treatment algorithm (Fig. 8.11) using the classification system proposed by Kuhn et al. [41].

A critical factor when selecting a suitable treatment strategy is to identify the patient's demand level (high or low), which is largely determined using the patient's age and activity level. However, patients who are physically active, employed, and living independently are typically assigned to the high demand group, regardless of age.

In fractures with a longitudinal line, fixation with two screws in the acromion generally results in satisfactory results, as there is no tension in the deltoid, deflecting the fragments inferiorly and generating impact into the joint (Fig. 8.12).

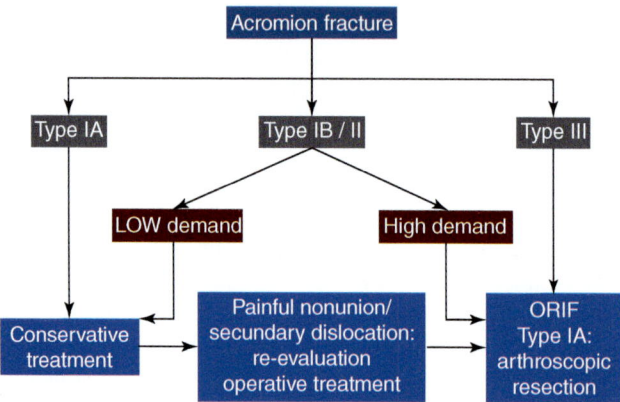

Fig. 8.11 Proposed treatment algorithm for acromion fractures by Hess et al. The classification is based on the original system described by Kuhn et al [45–47].

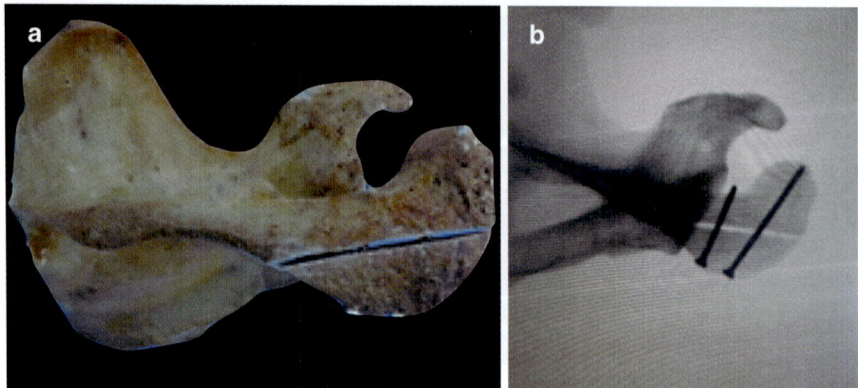

Fig. 8.12 (**a** and **b**): Simulation of fixation of an oblique fracture of the acromion with two lag screws

In cases of transverse or multifragmented fractures of the acromion, we use the posterior approach to the acromion with extension to the crest of the scapula. Our fixation strategy usually combines 3.5-, 2.7-, or 2.4-mm plates with lag or positioning screws out of the plate. If necessary, a suture augmentation can be placed to prevent secondary displacement (Figs. 8.13 and 8.14).

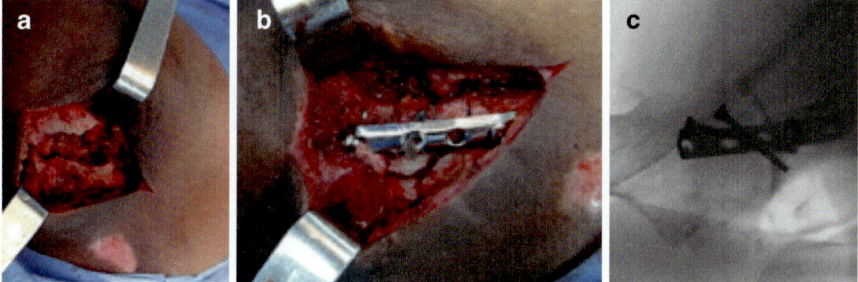

Fig. 8.13 (**a**) Intraoperative photograph showing the displaced acromion fracture. (**b**) Intraoperative photograph showing fracture reduction and fixation with plate and screws (one-third tubular plate with suture augmentation). (**c**) Postoperative fluoroscopy image showing adequate fracture reduction and fixation

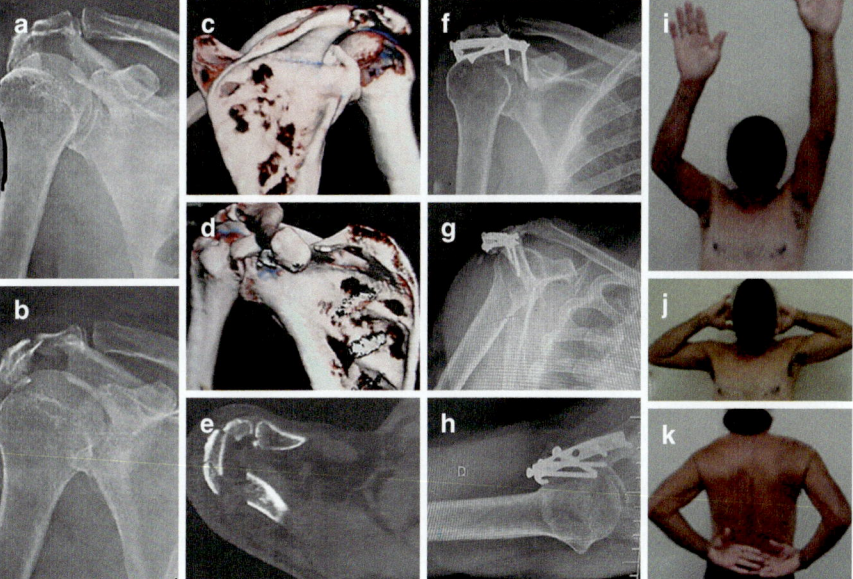

Fig. 8.14 (**a and b**) Radiographs of the shoulder showing a Kuhn et al. [18] type II multifragmentary fracture of the acromion extending to the most lateral part of the scapular spine. (**c–e**) Observe the amount of comminution on the CT scan. There is no obvious reduction of the subacromial space. (**f–h**) Fracture fixation was performed with a superiorly placed non-locked one-third tubular plate. (**i–k**) Observe the functional range of motion of the operated shoulder after fracture healing at 24 months postoperatively.

References

1. Gil JF, Haydar A. Isolated injury of the coracoid process: case report. J Trauma. 1991;31:1696–7.
2. Goss TP. Double disruptions of the superior shoulder suspensory complex. J Orthop Trauma. 1993;7:99–106.
3. Mulawka B, Jacobson A, Schroder L, et al. Triple and quadruple disruptions of the superior shoulder suspensory complex. J Orthop Trauma. 2015;29:264–70.
4. McGinnis M, Denton JR. Fractures of the scapula: a retrospective study of 40 fractured scapulae. J Trauma. 1989;29:1488–93.
5. Zlowodzki M, Bhandari M, Zelle BA, et al. Treatment of scapula fractures: systematic review of 520 fractures in 22 case series. J Orthop Trauma. 2006;20:230–3.
6. Lantry JM, Roberts CS, Giannoudis PV. Operative treatment of scapular fractures: a systematic review. Injury. 2008;39:271–83.
7. Ogawa K, Yoshida A, Takahashi M, et al. Fractures of the coracoid process. J Bone Joint Surg Br. 1997;79:17–9.
8. Rabbani GR, Cooper SM, Escobedo EM. An isolated coracoid fracture. Curr Probl Diagn Radiol. 2012;41:120–1.
9. Eyres KS, Brooks A, Stanley D. Fractures of the coracoid process. J Bone Joint Surg Br. 1995;77:425–8.
10. Li CH, Skalski MR, Matcuk GR Jr, et al. Coracoid process fractures: anatomy, injury patterns, multimodality imaging, and approach to management. Emergency Radiol. 2019;26:449–58.
11. Mohammed H, Skalski MR, Patel DB, Tomasian A, Schein AJ, White EA, GFR H III, Matcuk GR Jr. Coracoid process: the lighthouse of the shoulder. Radiographics. 2016;36(7):2084–101.
12. Alaia EF, Rosenberg ZS, Rossi I, et al. Growth plate injury at the base of the coracoid: MRI features. Skeletal Radiol. 2017;46(11):1507–12.
13. Knapik DM, Patel SH, Wetzel RJ, Voos JE. Prevalence and management of coracoid fracture sustained during sporting activities and time to return to sport: a systematic review. Am J Sports Med. 2018;46:753–8.
14. Kose O, Canbora K, Guler F, Kilicaslan OF, May H. Acromioclavicular dislocation associated with coracoid process fracture: report of two cases and review of the literature. Case Rep Orthop. 2015;2015:858969.
15. Wilson KM, Colwill JC. Combined acromioclavicular dislocation with coracoclavicular ligament disruption and coracoid process fracture. Am J Sports Med. 1989;17:697–8.
16. Li J, Sun W, Li GD, Li Q, Cai ZD. Fracture of the coracoid process associated with acromioclavicular dislocation: a case report. Orthopaedic Surg. 2010;2:165–7.
17. Protass JJ, Stampfli FV, Osmer JC. Coracoid process fracture diagnosis in acromioclavicular separation. Radiology. 1975;116(1):61–4.
18. Asbury S, Tennent TD. Avulsion fracture of the coracoid process: a case report. Injury. 2005;36:567–8.
19. Benton J, Nelson C. Avulsion of the coracoid process in an athlete. Report of a case. J Bone Joint Surg Am. 1971;53:356–8.
20. Boyer DWJ. Trapshooter's shoulder: stress fracture of the coracoid process. Case report. J Bone Joint Surg Am. 1975;57(6):862.
21. Bartoníček J, Tuček M, Strnad T, et al. Fractures of the coracoid process—pathoanatomy and classification: based on thirty nine cases with three dimensional computerised tomography reconstructions. Int Orthop. 2021;45(9):1009–15.
22. Chitre AR, Divecha HM, Hakimi M, et al. Traumatic isolated coracoid fractures in the adolescent. Case Rep Orthop. 2012;2012:371627.
23. Pedersen V, Prall WC, Ockert B, et al. Non-operative treatment of a fracture to the coracoid process with acromioclavicular dislocation in an adolescent. Orthop Rev. 2014;6:5499.
24. Thomas K, Ng VY, Bishop J. Nonoperative management of a sagittal coracoid fracture with a concomitant acromioclavicular joint separation. Int J Shoulder Surg. 2010;4:44–7.

25. Gross TP, Walcott ME. Rockwood and Matsen's the shoulder. 5th ed. Philadelphia: Elsevier; 2016.
26. Ogawa K, Ikegami H, Takeda T, Watanabe A. Defining impairment and treatment of subacute and chronic fractures of the coracoid process. J Trauma. 2009;67:1040–5.
27. Galvin JW, Kang J, Ma R, et al. Fractures of the coracoid process: evaluation, management, and outcomes. J Am Acad Orthop Surg. 2020;28:e706–15.
28. Hill BW, Jacobson AR, Anavian J, et al. Surgical management of coracoid fractures: technical tricks and clinical experience. J Orthop Trauma. 2014;28(5):e114–22.
29. Owens BD, Goss TP. The floating shoulder. J Bone Joint Surg (Br). 2006;88(11):1419–24.
30. Pires RE, Giordano V, Mendes de Souza FS, Labronici PJ. Current challenges and controversies in the management of scapular fractures: a review. Patient Saf Surg. 2021;15(6):1–18.
31. Ogawa K, Matsumura N, Ikegami H. Coracoid fractures: therapeutic strategy and surgical outcomes. J Trauma Acute Care Surg. 2012;72(2):E20–6.
32. Hardegger FH, Simpson LA, Weber BG. The operative treatment of scapular fractures. J Bone Joint Surg Br. 1984;66:725–31.
33. Wilber MC, Evans EB. Fractures of the scapula. An analysis of forty cases and a review of the literature. J Bone Joint Surg Am. 1977;59:358–62.
34. Bauer G, Fleischmann W, Dussler E. Displaced scapular fractures: indication and long-term results of open reduction and internal fixation. Arch Orthop Trauma Surg. 1995;114:215–9.
35. McGahan JP, Rab GT, Dublin A. Fractures of the scapula. J Trauma. 1980;20:880–8.
36. McGahan JP, Rab GT. Fracture of the acromion associated with an axillary nerve deficit: a case report and review of the literature. Clin Orthop Rel Res. 1980;147:216–8.
37. Gorczyca JT, Davis RT, Hartford JM, et al. Open reduction internal fixation after displacement of a previously nondisplaced acromial fracture in a multiply injured patient: case report and review of literature. J Orthop Trauma. 2001;15(5):369–73.
38. Harris RD, Harris JH. The prevalence and significance of missed scapular fractures in blunt chest trauma. Am J Roentgenol. 1988;151:747–50.
39. Ryu RKN, Fan RSP, Dunbar WHV. The treatment of symptomatic os acromiale. Orthopedics. 1999;22:325–8.
40. Ogawa K, Naniwa T. Fractures of the acromion and the lateral scapular spine. J Shoulder Elb Surg. 1997;6:544–8.
41. Kuhn JE, Blasier RB, Carpenter JE. Fractures of the acromion process: a proposed classification system. J Orthop Trauma. 1994;8:6–13.
42. Belien H, Biesmans H, Steenwerckx A, et al. Prebending of osteosynthesis plate using 3D printed models to treat symptomatic os acromiale and acromial fracture. J Exp Orthop. 2017;4(1):34.
43. Kim DS, Yoon YS, Kang DH. Comparison of early fixation and delayed reconstruction after displacement in previously nondisplaced acromion fractures. Orthopedics. 2010;33:392.
44. Hess F, Zettl R, Welter J, et al. The traumatic acromion fracture: review of the literature, clinical examples, and proposal of a treatment algorithm. Arch Orthop Trauma Surg. 2019;139:651–8.
45. Anavian J, Wijdicks CA, Schroder LK, et al. Surgery for scapula process fractures: good outcome in 26 patients. Acta Orthop. 2009;80:344–50.
46. Hill BW, Anavian J, Jacobson AR, et al. Surgical management of isolated acromion fractures: technical tricks and clinical experience. J Orthop Trauma. 2014;28:e107–13.
47. Ringelberg JA. EMG and force production of some human shoulder muscles during isometric abduction. J Biomech. 1985;18:939–47.

Chapter 9
Special Considerations: The Floating Shoulder—Myths and Reality

Fabio A. Suarez Romero and Federico Suarez Rodriguez

9.1 Introduction

The recent increase in the incidence of scapular fractures may be due to a shift into a more physically active population, the practice of extreme sports, and jobs that are physically demanding. Non-operative treatment has generally been the treatment of choice. However, the experience has shown that, depending on the degree and type of displacement, non-operative treatment is usually followed by residual pain and functional impairment. Furthermore, the scarcity in the literature and the lack of consensus about pathomechanics make it difficult to standardize a treatment protocol [1–3].

9.2 Definition

Floating shoulder is defined as an ipsilateral glenoid neck and clavicle fracture and to a lesser extent, an associated coracoclavicular and/or coracoacromial ligament injury. The double disruption of the SSSC plays a key role in the floating shoulder [4, 5].

F. A. Suarez Romero (✉)
Department of Orthopedics and Upper Extremity Surgery, Universidad Militar Nueva Granada, Hospital Militar Central, Bogotá, Colombia

F. Suarez Rodriguez
School of Medicine, Universidad Militar Nueva Granada, Bogotá, Colombia

© The Author(s), under exclusive license to Springer Nature Switzerland AG 2024
R. E. Pires et al. (eds.), *Fractures of the Scapula*,
https://doi.org/10.1007/978-3-031-58498-5_9

Ganz and Noesberger [1] initially described this traumatic scenario as the combination of a scapula and a clavicle fracture or an acromioclavicular dislocation along with complete rupture of the coracoclavicular ligaments.

Herscovici et al. [2] introduced later the concept of the "floating shoulder" characterized by the ipsilateral fractures of the neck of the scapula and the middle third of the clavicle.

Several authors have defined the floating shoulder as the fracture of the surgical neck of the scapula, the complete rupture of the coracoclavicular ligaments, and a clavicle fracture just medial to the footprint of insertion of the coracoclavicular ligaments [1–5].

The association of a midshaft clavicle with a scapular body fracture is frequently misinterpreted as a floating shoulder. This injury pattern presents no influence on stability or displacement of the glenoid neck. Therefore, fixation of the clavicle only generally does not result in improvement of the scapular displacement [6].

9.3 Anatomy

9.3.1 Superior Shoulder Suspensory Complex

The superior shoulder suspensory complex is an osteofibrous ring formed by the glenoid cavity, the coracoid process, the coracoacromial and coracoclavicular ligaments, the lateral third of the clavicle, the acromioclavicular joint, and the acromion [4].

The superior part is the middle third of the clavicle, and the inferior part is the junction of the most lateral portion of the scapular body and the most medial portion of the glenoid neck.

The superior shoulder suspensory complex consists of 3 units:

1. The clavicular- acromioclavicular joint-acromion (Fig. 9.1).
2. The clavicular-coracoclavicular ligaments and coracoid linkage.
3. The junction of the glenoid, coracoid, and acromion with the scapular body (the three process-scapular body junction) [5].

This complex maintains a normal stable relationship between the scapula, the upper extremity, and the axial skeleton. It also allows limited motion via the acromioclavicular joint and the coracoclavicular ligament and provides a firm attachment point for several soft-tissue structures (Fig. 9.2).

Some surgeons have adopted Goss's concept, in the sense of describing floating shoulder as injuries with involvement of the superior shoulder suspensory complex at more than two levels [7, 8].

Fig. 9.1 Illustration of the anatomy of the superior shoulder suspensory complex

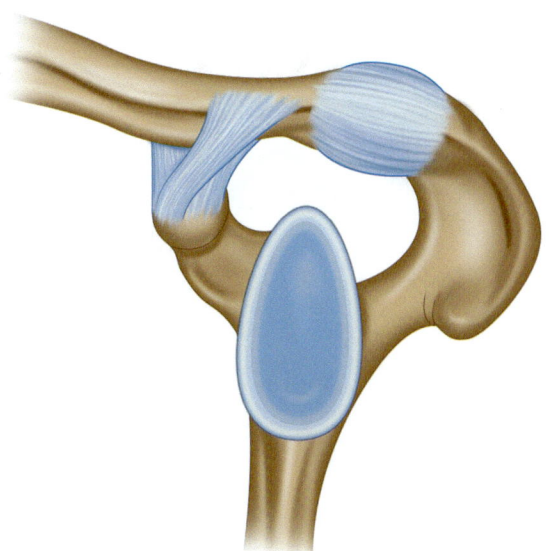

The coracoid process along with the coracoclavicular and coracoacromial ligaments, the pectoralis minor, the short head of the biceps brachii, and the coracobrachialis play a significant role in this traumatic injury. An avulsion at the base of the coracoid process compromises the stabilization effect of the coracoclavicular and coracoacromial ligaments. This neutralizes the pulling deforming force of the muscles that take attachment points on the coracoid process. In those instances, when there is disruption of both, the coracoclavicular and coracoacromial ligaments, these muscles pull the glenoid distal and medially. A truly unstable scenario finds a fracture of the acromial apex and a rupture of the coracoclavicular ligament with a comminuted fracture of the lateral end of the clavicle. This pattern causes a separation of the fragments both from the clavicle shaft and the acromioclavicular joint.

We cannot overlook the functional relevance of the connection between the scapula and the axial skeleton. The trapezius, rhomboid, anterior serratus, and scapula elevator maintain the stability of the thoracoscapular interface. They control the relationship between the scapular spine, acromion, and acromioclavicular joint with the chest wall. It is also important to keep in mind that the trapezius muscle attaches to the scapula when reducing the fracture fragments and that the rotator cuffs insertion onto the proximal humerus reflects on the stability and valgus displacement of the glenoid fragment (Fig. 9.3).

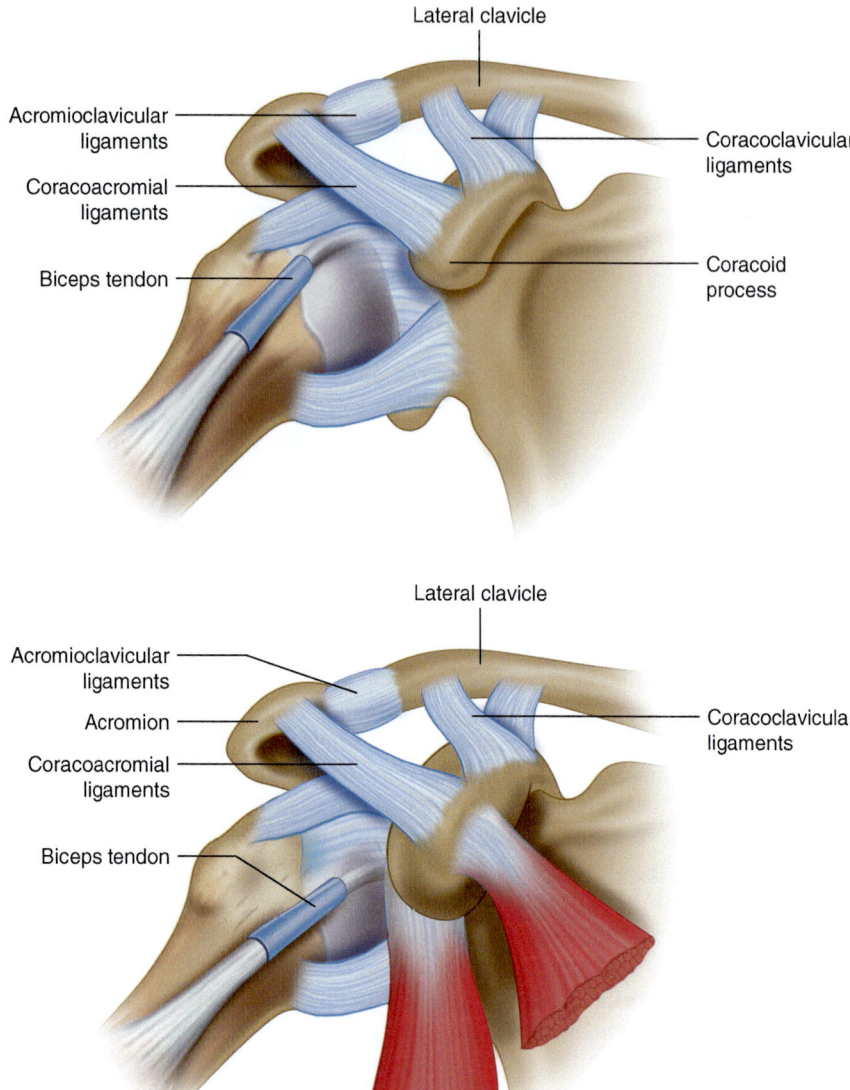

Fig. 9.2 Illustration of the anatomy of the superior shoulder suspensory complex. *A* Acromion, *BT* Biceps tendon, *AC* Acromioclavicular ligaments, *CA* Coracoacromial ligaments, *CP* Coracoid process, *CC* Coracoclavicular ligaments, *LC* Lateral clavicle

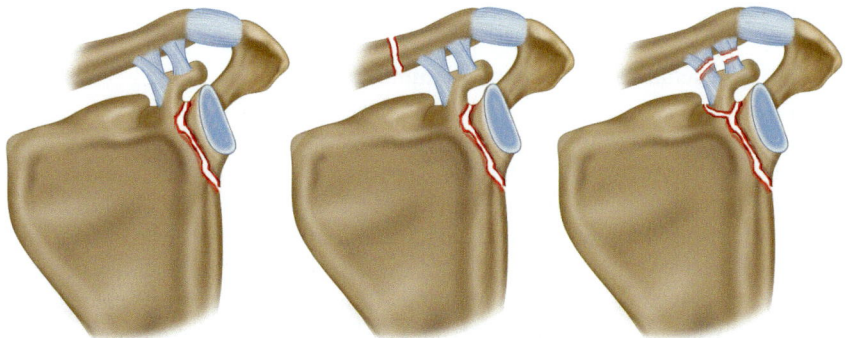

Fig. 9.3 Illustration of a glenoid neck fracture and the degree of instability caused by associate injuries of the SSSC

9.4 Surgical Indications

Currently, there is no consensus on absolute indications for surgical fixation. This can be credited, at least in part, to the difficulty in a precise definition of this traumatic injury [9, 10]. In addition, factors like the surgeon's preference, the level of patient activity, and associated injuries make the decision process even more challenging. In general, non-displaced or minimally displaced fractures are amenable for non-operative management. On the other hand, among the suggested surgical indications, one can include a scapular neck fracture with significant displacement: ≥ 1 cm of translational displacement of the glenoid fragment, $\geq 40°$ of angular displacement of the glenoid fragment (either on the sagittal or coronal planes), and a glenopolar angle (GPA) $<20°$ [11, 12].

A systematic review [13] found no significant differences in terms of functional outcomes when comparing non-surgical treatment, clavicle fracture fixation alone, and surgical fixation of both the clavicle and scapular fractures. A stable and reliable fixation might allow for an expedited rehabilitation program hence decreasing the chance of shoulder stiffness.

The floating flail chest, a new described entity, is another potential indication for double fixation (clavicle and scapula) in patients with associated floating shoulder and flail chest. In a case series of 41 patients presenting association of floating shoulder and flail chest, Cunninghan et al. [14] compared 23 treated with operative stabilization and 18 treated non-operatively. The authors reported that the restoration of the scapula-clavicular arch unloads of the flail chest and improves pain control and respiratory function, thereby decreasing duration of mechanical ventilation and intensive care unit length of stay.

9.4.1 Surgical Approaches

9.4.1.1 Clavicular Approach and Fixation

This approach is used through a standard anterior incision parallel and just inferior to the anteroinferior edge of the clavicle. The supraclavicular nerves should be identified and protected throughout the entire procedure (Fig. 9.4). A scalpel or periosteal elevator is used for deeper dissection. Careful manipulation of small fragments is required to avoid compromise of their vascular supply and potential necrosis. Joysticks or pointed clamps become useful for handling lateral and medial fragments during the reduction maneuvers, especially in the presence of shortening. In addition, a mini-distractor can help with length restoration and fragment organization (Fig. 9.5). If the intermediate fragment allows, a lag screw or minifragment plates may be used to optimize reduction and construct stability.

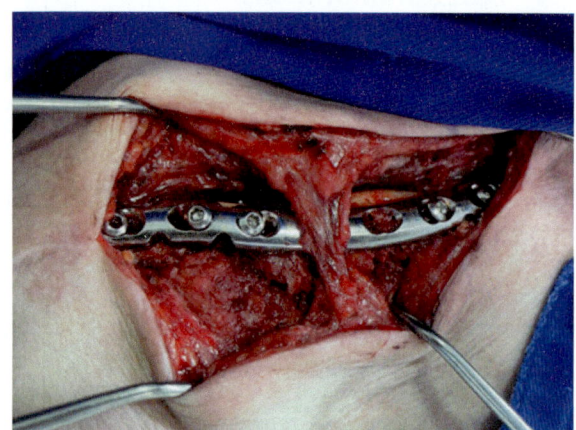

Fig. 9.4 Intraoperative photograph showing identification and protection of the supraclavicular nerves during the surgical procedure

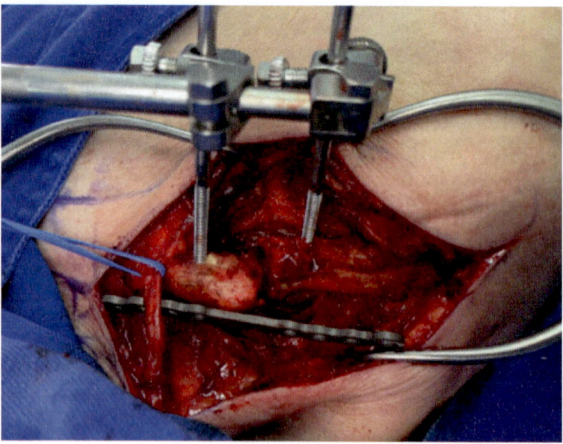

Fig. 9.5 Intraoperative photograph showing a mini-distractor applied to the clavicle to achieve length restoration

Once the reduction is achieved, the plate is positioned either on the superior aspect (author's preference) or on the anterior edge. With the anterior placement, the plate needs to be contoured; this location is more demanding, but safer. Moreover, longer screws can be applied when the plate is inserted on the anterior surface of the clavicle. The decision to use either locking vs standard cortical screws depends on the bone quality, fracture pattern, and required stiffness. Nowadays, precontoured "s" plates are available to expedite surgical procedures. Radiographic evaluation of the glenoid is mandatory to assess its involvement and the potential need for fixation.

9.4.1.2 Scapular Approach and Fixation

The patient is either placed in a lateral or prone position. The author's preference is lateral decubitus to make possible the exposure and fixation of the clavicle and the scapula (Fig. 9.6). However, if the clavicle fracture is located in the medial third of the bone, fixing the clavicle in lateral positioning may be extremely challenging. This position is also used in patients with pulmonary compromise. It is important to keep in mind that, with the lateral positioning, and depending on the scapular fracture pattern, it is difficult to correct the medialization of the glenoid due to the pressure exerted by the arm.

For the glenoid, the standard Judet [15] or the modified Judet [16] approaches offer satisfactory visualization of the medial and lateral pillars of the scapula. The landmarks for these approaches are the spine of the scapula, the medial border, and the glenoid fossa. The skin incision starts on the posterolateral corner of the acromion. This incision is performed in line with the subcutaneous spine of the scapula and curved inferiorly in line with the medial border until reaching the inferior angle of the scapula. The posterior deltoid insertion and the acromion are exposed. The posterior deltoid is bluntly detached from the posterior spine of the scapula. Caution must be focused on preventing excessive inferior traction under the teres minor to

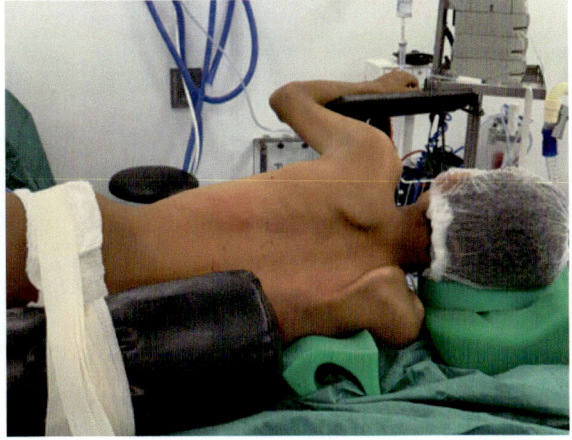

Fig. 9.6 Lateral positioning for floating shoulder fixation

protect the axillary nerve. If a classic Judet [15] approach is performed, the infraspinatus muscle is completely detached from the posterior aspect of the scapula. Preserving a flap for final reinsertion, the infraspinatus muscle is detached from the medial border, from the spine, and completely elevated from the infraspinatus fossa. The entire muscle can be elevated in a subperiosteal fashion to prevent neurovascular compromise of the suprascapular nerve (Fig. 9.7a). The modified Judet [16] approach exposes the medial border, the body, the inferior aspect of the spine, the base of the acromion, and the neck of the scapula. The lateral window is developed between the teres minor and the infraspinatus muscles. A window on the medial edge of the scapula may be useful to fix the medial scapula component.

9.4.1.3 Reduction Instruments and Implants for Fracture Fixation

Ideally, the surgical fixation should be performed acutely. However, in the presence of associated injuries such as thoracic, pulmonary, and spine injuries, this would need to be delayed ensuring respiratory and clinical support. Special reduction strategies may be necessary with the use of Schanz screws as a joystick, ball spike pushers, pointed clamps, and mini-distractors. The strongest structure offered by the lateral and medial pillars and the base of the spine are the most appropriate places for implant's placement (Fig. 9.7b).

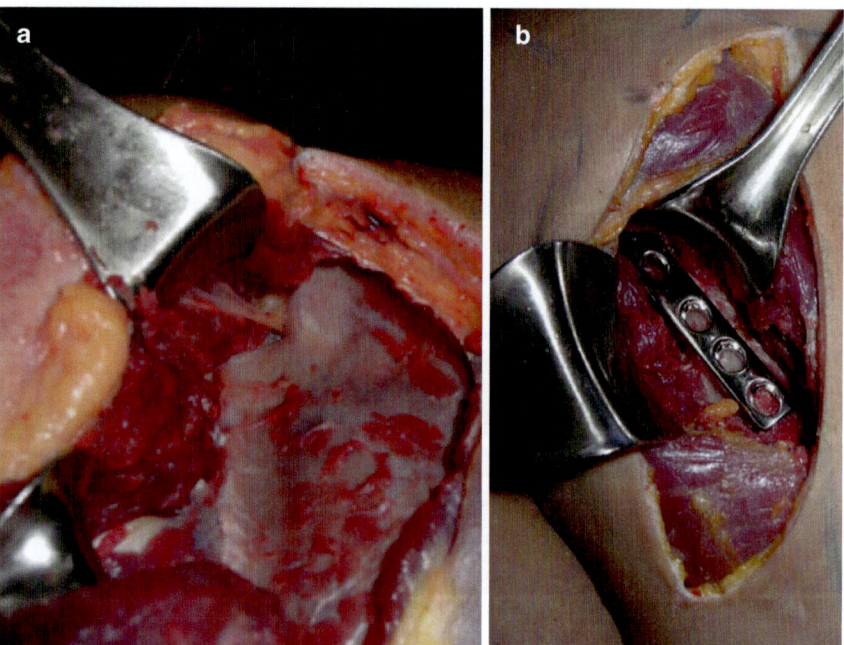

Fig. 9.7 (**a**): Classic Judet approach with exposure of the suprascapular nerve. (**b**): Intraoperative photograph showing the lateral window and plate placement to fix the lateral pillar of the scapula

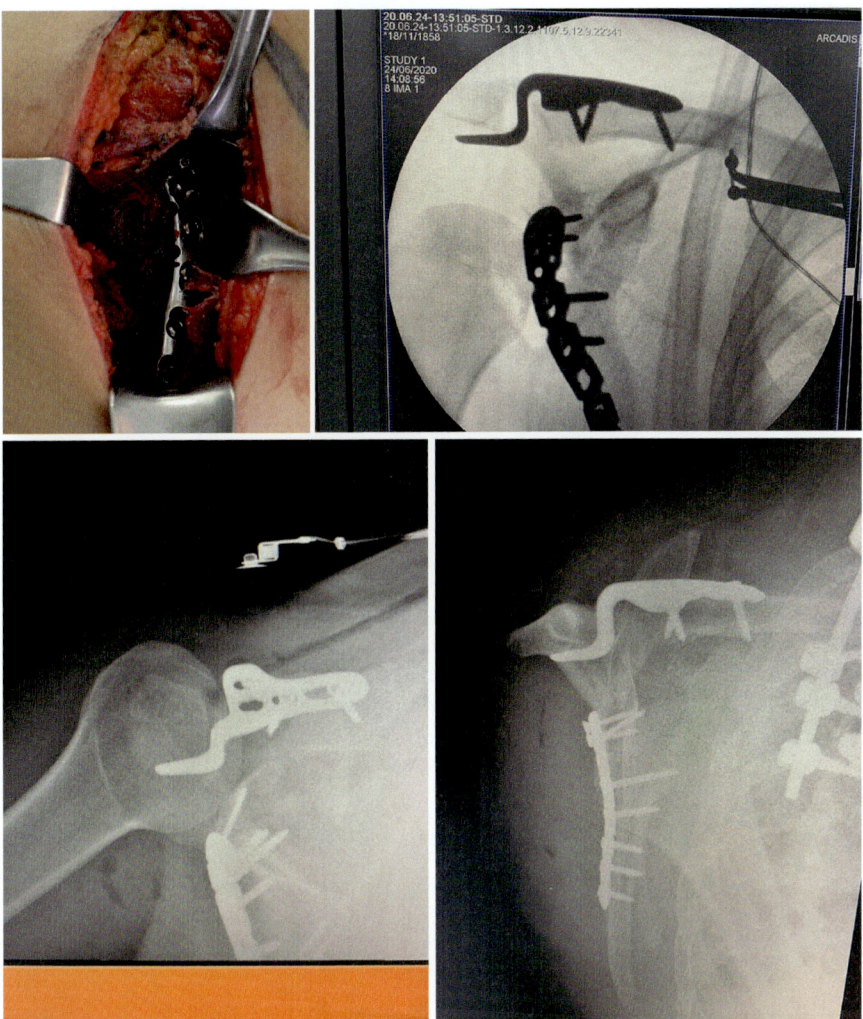

Fig. 9.8 Fixation of the lateral pillar of the scapula with the off label use of a distal clavicle plate

Conventional 2.7, 3.5 mm reconstruction plates or 2.7, 3.5 mm LCP plates are used to fix the lateral and medial scapular edges. Scapular spine fractures are preferable fixed with 2.7 mm minifragment plates. However, depending on the size of the bone, they can be occasionally fixed using 3.5 mm reconstruction plates. If available, precontoured clavicle plates may be an interesting option although in off label use to the scapula (Fig. 9.8). The hook clavicle plate may be used in cases with acromioclavicular dislocation or terminal fractures in the distal end of the clavicle.

9.5 Complications

The involvement of the superior shoulder suspensory complex causes an unstable situation and can generate poor outcomes with the development of non-union or malunion, subacromial dysfunction, subacromial impingement, weakness, discomfort and muscular fatigue, frozen shoulder, shoulder deformity, failed fixation, neurovascular involvement with a dropped shoulder, and arthrosis. In the presence of high-energy trauma, there is an increase in the incidence of associated injuries such as brachial plexus, cervical spine, and thoracic fractures [6–17].

9.6 Conclusions

Floating shoulder is a relatively uncommon injury, with significant controversy and debate in special regarding the treatment options. Non-operative and operative management appear to provide adequate outcomes in appropriately individualized patients. Proper reduction and double fixation (scapula and clavicle) usually provide adequate stabilization of the SSSC and restoration of the glenopolar angle, which are the goals of treatment of the floating shoulder. Although a floating shoulder with non-displaced or minimally displaced scapular fracture may be safely treated with clavicle fixation only, the exact amount of displacement is still a source of controversy in the literature [7, 18–22]. The rehabilitation protocol is thoroughly detailed in a special chapter of this book.

References

1. Ganz R, Noesberger B. Treatment of scapular fractures. Hefte Unfallheilkd. 1975;126(126):59–62. German
2. Herscovici D Jr, Fiennes AGTW, Allgöwer M, Rüedi TP. The floating shoulder: ipsilateral clavicle and scapular neck fractures. J Bone Joint Surg Br. 1992;74(3):362–4.
3. Leung KS, Lam TP. Open reduction and internal fixation of ipsilateral fractures of the scapular neck and clavicle. J Bone Joint Surg Am. 1993;75(7):1015–8.
4. Mulawka B, Jacobson AR, Schroder LK, Cole PA. Triple and quadruple disruptions of the superior shoulder suspensory complex. J Orthop Trauma. 2015;29(6):264–70.
5. Goss TP. Double disruptions of the superior shoulder suspensory complex. J Orthop Trauma. 1993;7(2):99–106.
6. Bartonicek J, Tucek M, Nanka O. Floating shoulder: myths and reality. JBJS Rev. 2018;6(10):e5.
7. Lin TL, Li YF, Hsu CJ, Hung CH, Lin CC, Fong YC, Hsu HC, Tsai CH. Clinical outcome and radiographic change of ipsilateral scapular neck and clavicular shaft fracture: comparison of operation and conservative treatment. J Orthop Surg Res. 2015;28(10):9–16.
8. Oh W, Jeon IH, Kyung S, Park C, Kim T, Ihn C. The treatment of double disruption of the superior shoulder suspensory complex. Int Orthop. 2002;26(3):145–9.
9. Herscovici D Jr. Open reduction and internal fixation of ipsilateral fractures of the scapular neck and clavicle. J Bone Joint Surg Am. 1994;76(7):1112–3.

10. Oh CW, Kyung HS, Kim PT, Ihn JC. Failure of internal fixation of the clavicle in the treatment of ipsilateral clavicle and glenoid neck fractures. J Orthop Sci. 2001;6(6):601–3.
11. van Noort A, te Slaa RL, Marti RK, van der Werken C. The floating shoulder. A multicentre study. J Bone Joint Surg Br. 2001;83(6):795–8.
12. Morey VM, Chua KHZ, Ng ZD, Tan HMB, Kumar VP. Management of the floating shoulder: does the glenopolar angle influence outcomes? A systematic review. Orthop Traumatol Surg Res. 2018;104(1):53–8.
13. Dombrowsky AR, Boudreau S, Quade J, Brabston EW, Ponce BA, Momaya AM. Clinical outcomes following conservative and surgical management of floating shoulder injuries: a systematic review. J Shoulder Elb Surg. 2020;29(3):634–42.
14. Cunningham BP, Bosch L, Swanson D, McLemore R, Rhorer AS, Parikh HR, Albersheim M, Ortega G. The floating flail chest: acute management of an injury combination of the floating shoulder and flail chest. J Orthop Trauma Rehab. 2020;27(1):10–5.
15. Judet R. Traitement chirurgical des fractures de l'omoplate. Acta Orthop Belg. 1964;30:673–8.
16. Obremskey WT, Lyman JR. A modified Judet approach to the scapula. J Orthop Trauma. 2004;18(10):696–9.
17. Pires RE, Giordano V, Mendes de Souza FS, Labronici PJ. Current challenges and controversies in the management of scapular fractures: a review. Patient Saf Surg. 2021;15(6):1–18.
18. Kim KC, Rhee KJ, Shin HD, Yang JY. Can the glenopolar angle be used to predict outcome and treatment of the floating shoulder? J Trauma. 2008;64(1):174–8.
19. Yadav V, Khare GN, Singh S, Kumaraswamy V, Sharma N, Rai AK, Ramaswamy AG, Sharma H. A prospective study comparing conservative with operative treatment in patients with a 'floating shoulder' including assessment of the prognostic value of the glenopolar angle. Bone Joint J. 2013;95-B(6):815–9.
20. Pailhes RG, Bonnevialle N, Laffosse J, Tricoire J, Cavaignac E, Chiron P. Floating shoulders: clinical and radiographic analysis at a mean follow-up of 11 years. Int J Shoulder Surg. 2013;7(2):59–64.
21. Gilde AK, Hoffmann MF, Sietsema DL, Jones CB. Functional outcomes of operative fixation of clavicle fractures in patients with floating shoulder girdle injuries. J Orthop Traumatol. 2015;16(3):221–7.
22. Cole PA, Gauger EM, Schroder LK. Management of scapular fractures. J Am Acad Orthop Surg. 2012;20(3):130–41.

Chapter 10
Special Considerations: The Floating Flail Chest—A New Entity

Robinson Esteves Pires, Vincenzo Giordano, and Pedro José Labronici

10.1　Floating Flail Chest—A New Entity

The definition of floating shoulder remains controversial. Ganz and Noesberger [1], in 1975, firstly described the "floating shoulder" as an injury consisting of ipsilateral clavicle and glenoid neck fractures. Goss [2] was responsible for expanding the understanding of this injury and recognizing the role of ligamentous on the disruption of the superior shoulder suspensory complex.

Although some authors [3–5] described the presence of floating shoulder when two or more structures of the superior shoulder suspensory complex are disrupted, Bartoníček et al. [6] postulate that floating shoulder is an unstable displaced fracture of the anatomical or surgical glenoid neck of the scapula in association or not with a clavicle fracture. The authors also highlighted that, in cases of surgical neck fractures of the scapula, there must occur an associated rupture of both the coracoacromial and coracoclavicular ligaments or a fracture of their osseous-equivalent structures (extra-articular or intra- or extra-articular coracoid base and acromion). It is noteworthy that the combination of a midshaft clavicle fracture with a scapular body fracture, generally an infraglenoid fracture of the scapular body, is frequently misinterpreted as a floating shoulder. This injury pattern presents no influence on stability or displacement of the glenoid neck. Therefore, isolated fixation of the clavicle fracture usually does not result in improvement of the scapula displacement [6].

R. E. Pires (✉)
Department of the Locomotor Apparatus, Federal University of Minas Gerais, Belo Horizonte, Minas Gerais, Brazil

V. Giordano
Orthopedics Department, Hospital Municipal Miguel Couto, Rio de Janeiro, Brazil

P. J. Labronici
Department of General and Specialized Surgery, Fluminense Federal University, Niterói, Brazil

© The Author(s), under exclusive license to Springer Nature Switzerland AG 2024
R. E. Pires et al. (eds.), *Fractures of the Scapula*, https://doi.org/10.1007/978-3-031-58498-5_10

Figure 10.1 shows the treatment of a 53-year-old polytraumatized patient who presented chest trauma and associated clavicle fracture and infraglenoid fracture of the scapular body. Figure 10.2 shows the result of another polytrauma patient who underwent open reduction and fracture fixation for combined scapula and clavicle fractures. Even though some improvement of the glenopolar angle compared pre- and postoperatively was reported after isolated fixation of the clavicle, we do not routinely observe such improvement in clinical practice, which we believe can be attributed to associated capsuloligamentous injuries of the superior shoulder suspensory complex [7].

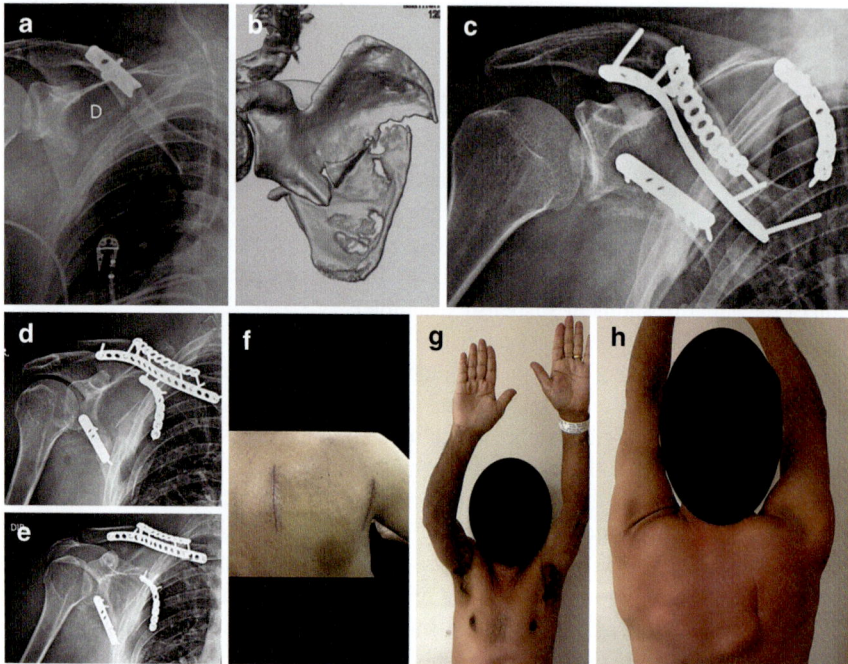

Fig. 10.1 A 53-year-old patient was hit by a truck while riding a bicycle. He suffered polytrauma with severe blunt chest trauma and associated clavicle and infraglenoid fracture of the scapula body. Observe that the patient previously presented a clavicle shaft fracture that was treated with open reduction and internal fixation. Treatment included open reduction and internal fixation of the clavicle with double plating, associated with minimally invasive fixation of the scapula body. Observe the clinical result of the patient after fracture healing. (**a** and **b**) Radiograph in anteroposterior view and 3D CT of the shoulder showing associated clavicle and infraglenoid fracture of the scapula body. (**c–e**) Postoperative radiographs showing open reduction and fracture fixation with plate and screws. (**f–h**) Photographs of the clinical results after fracture healing

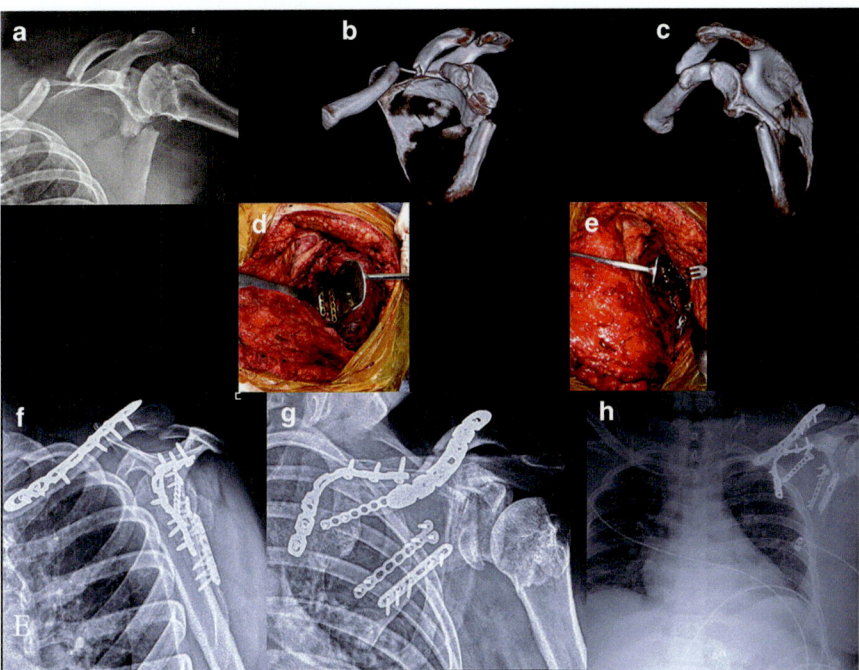

Fig. 10.2 (**a–c**) Radiograph and 3D-CT reconstruction of the left shoulder in anteroposterior view of a 24-year-old male patient who suffered a car accident and presented a severely displaced midshaft clavicle fracture in combination with an infraglenoidal fracture of the scapula body. Observe that the patient presented a sequela of previous proximal humeral and glenoid fractures, with no residual shoulder instability. (**d** and **e**) Perioperative photographs showing the modified Judet approach. Observe the fixation of the lateral pillar of the scapula with two plates at the interval between the infraspinatus and teres minor muscles (**d**). The medial pillar of the scapula was reduced and fixed with a twisted reconstruction locking plate (**e**). (**f–h**) Radiographs showing fracture healing after 3 months post-surgery. No clinical instability was observed in the postoperative evaluation

The treatment of floating shoulder also remains a topic of debate. While some authors advocate non-operative treatment, others defend isolated fixation of the clavicle, while a third group recommends the fixation of both scapula and clavicle (Figs. 10.3 and 10.4) [8–11]. Figure 10.5 shows a bilateral scapula fracture in a patient who suffered a motorcycle accident.

Rib fractures occur in up to 73% of floating shoulder cases [12]. The most severe type of chest wall injury has been described as a flail chest [13–23]. The definition of flail chest has been controversial in the literature, being recently defined as fractures of three or more consecutive ribs, with each rib fractured in two or more places [11]. This phenomenon of a free segment of the chest wall clinically results in

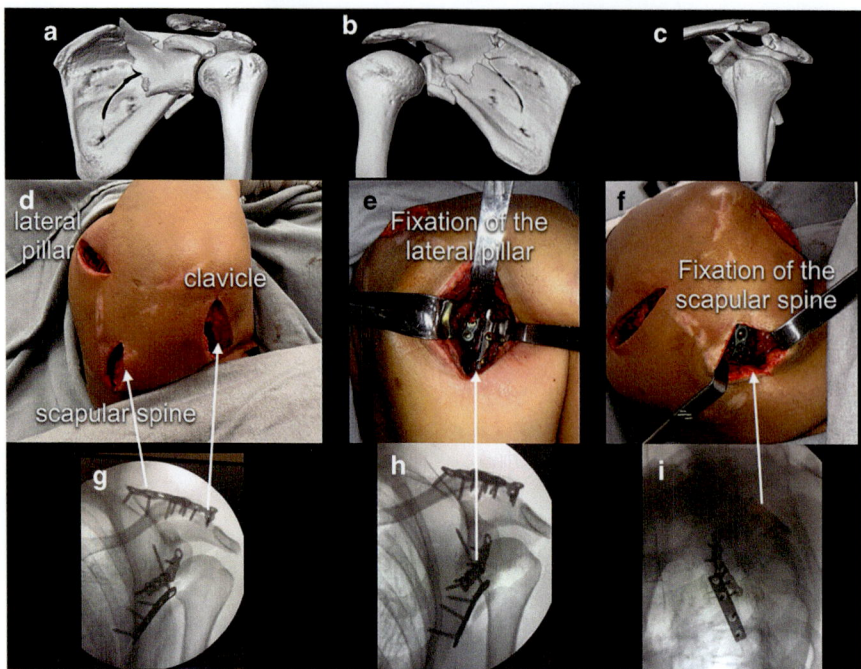

Fig. 10.3 A 28-year-old male patient suffered a motorcycle accident and presented a floating shoulder. (**a–c**) 3D-CT showing the associated clavicle, scapula neck, and scapula spine fracture. (**d–f**) Perioperative photographs showing three minimally invasive windows used for fracture fixation. (**g–i**) Perioperative fluoroscopy images showing fracture reduction and fixation of the clavicle, scapula spine, and scapula neck using 2.8 mm locking plates

paradoxical breathing, which hinders adequate toilet of pulmonary secretions. The incidence of flail chest was reported to be greater than 6% in patients with blunt chest trauma [11, 13, 14]. Mortality of the flail chest has been reported to reach 33% [15, 16]. Current Eastern Association for the Surgery of Trauma guidelines favor non-operative management of flail chest [17, 18]. Nevertheless, a cohort and two randomized studies presented improved outcomes with surgical treatment in selected patients [18–20].

Cunningham et al. [11] were the first to introduce the new entity "floating flail chest." In a case series of 41 patients presenting association of floating shoulder and flail chest, the authors compared 23 patients treated with operative stabilization and 18 treated non-operatively. The authors reported that the restoration of the scapula-clavicular arch unloads of the flail chest and improves pain control and respiratory function, thereby decreasing duration of mechanical ventilation days and intensive care unit length of stay (Fig. 10.6). Our treatment protocol for floating shoulder is the isolated fixation of the clavicle fracture, if the scapular neck presents no displacement or minimal displacement and the CT with 3D reconstruction GP angle in neutral rotation is >22° (Fig. 10.7).

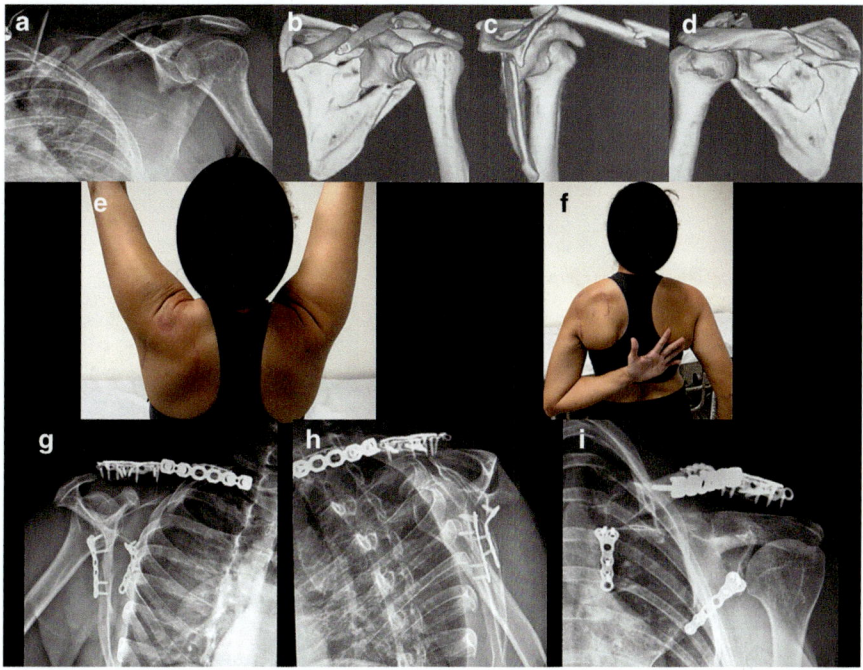

Fig. 10.4 A 34-year-old female patient suffered a bicycle accident and presented a segmental fracture of the clavicle, associated with a complex fracture of the scapula (scapular neck and spine). (**a–d**) Radiograph and 3D CT showing the associated clavicle and scapula fractures. (**e** and **f**) Postoperative photographs after fracture healing. Observe the two windows used for fixation of the scapular fracture. (**g–i**) Postoperative radiographs after fracture healing

Otherwise, we fix both clavicle and scapula, starting our fixation with the clavicle, in a beach chair or horizontal position. After clavicle fixation, we place the patient lateral to perform scapula fixation, either using the modified Judet approach or preferably a combination of minimally invasive approaches. Prone positioning should be avoided in patients with severe pulmonary trauma. Considering floating shoulder flail chest patients, we currently consider restoration of the scapula-clavicular arch, fixing both clavicle and scapula (Fig. 10.8).

The literature is still controversy regarding surgical indications for rib fractures, although some authors advocate fixing rib fractures for carefully selected patients with multiple rib fractures or flail chest [19, 21–26]. Chuang et al. [27] reported that for concomitant and ipsilateral scapula and multiple rib fractures that meet the surgical indications, the mirror Judet approach can be a safe and effective treatment option, since it allows for adequate fixation of both fractures (ribs and scapula) and provides acceptable functional outcomes in well-selected patients.

The postoperative care is almost the same described for glenoid neck and body scapula fractures and is outlined in detail in Chap. 13. The unique difference lies on the need of a special attention for the clearance of pulmonary secretions and improvement of lung function.

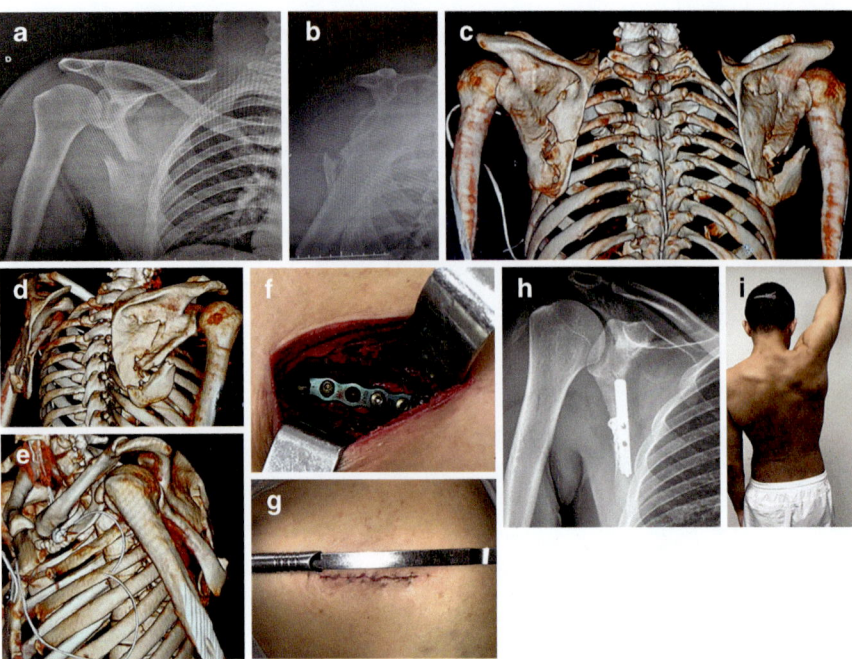

Fig. 10.5 Fig. 10.5 shows a bilateral scapula fracture in a patient who suffered a motorcycle accident. (**a–e**) Radiograph and 3D-CT showing the bilateral scapular fracture. Note the decrease of the glenopolar angle on the right side. (**f** and **g**) Perioperative (**f**) and postoperative (**g**) photographs showing the minimally invasive fixation of the lateral pillar of the scapula with double plating. (**h**): Postoperative radiograph of the right shoulder showing fracture reduction and fixation with plate and screws. (**i**) Photograph of the clinical result after 2 weeks postoperatively. Observe the active movement of the shoulder

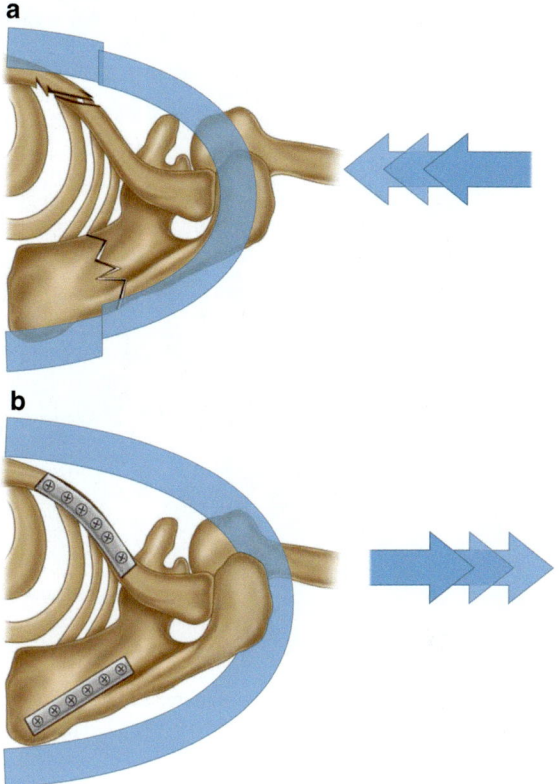

Fig. 10.6 (**a**, **b**) Illustration depicting the restoration of the scapula-clavicular arch in a floating flail chest scenario after clavicle and scapula fixation

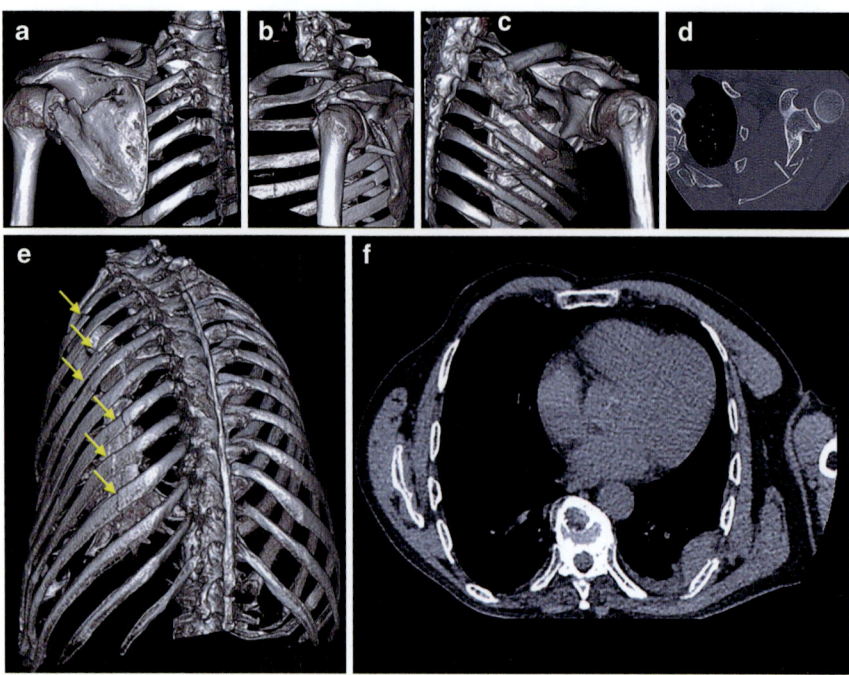

Fig. 10.7 A 70-year-old male patient suffered a high-energy chest trauma and presented a floating flail chest. (**a–f**) CT scan showing the associated clavicle, scapula, and multiple rib fractures (observe the yellow arrows depicting the rib fractures)

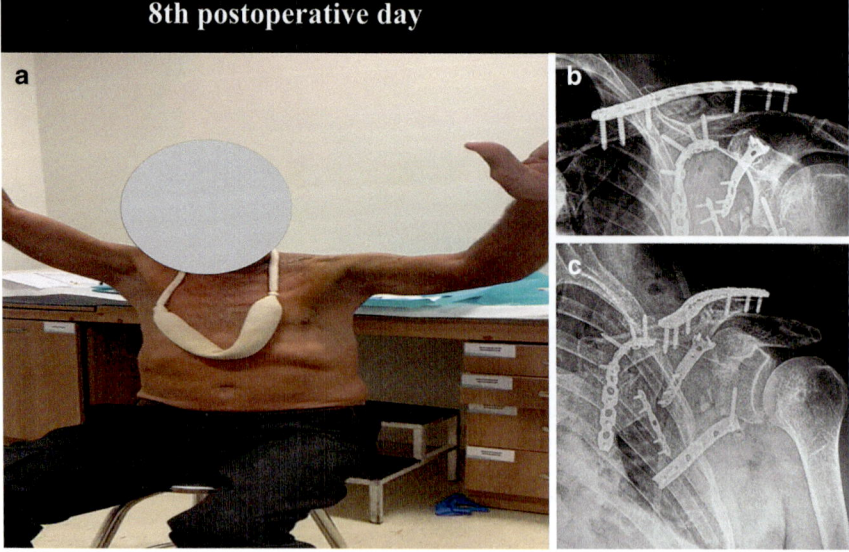

Fig. 10.8 (**a**) Observe the clinical aspect of the patient after 8 days of fracture fixation of both clavicle and scapula, with restoration of the scapula-clavicular arch. (**b** and **c**) Postoperative radiographs showing fracture reduction and fixation with plate and screws through the classic Judet approach

References

1. Ganz R, Noesberger B. Treatment of scapular fractures. Hefte Unfallheilkd. 1975;126:59–62. [Article in German].
2. Goss TP. Scapular fractures and dislocations: diagnosis and treatment. J Am Acad Orthop Surg. 1995;3(1):22–33.
3. Oh W, Jeon IH, Kyung S, Park C, Kim T, Ihn C. The treatment of double disruption of the superior shoulder suspensory complex. Int Orthop. 2002;26(3):145–9.
4. Mulawka B, Jacobson AR, Schroder LK, Cole PA. Triple and quadruple disruptions of the superior shoulder suspensory complex. J Orthop Trauma. 2015;29(6):264–70.
5. Goss TP. Double disruptions of the superior shoulder suspensory complex. J Orthop Trauma. 1993;7(2):99–106.
6. Bartoníček J, Tuček M, Naňka O. Floating shoulder: myths and reality. JBJS Rev. 2018;6(10):e5.
7. Kim KC, Rhee KJ, Shin HD, Yang JY. Can the glenopolar angle be used to predict outcome and treatment of the floating shoulder? J Trauma. 2008;64(1):174–8.
8. Edwards SG, Whittle AP, Wood GW 2nd. Nonoperative treatment of ipsilateral fractures of the scapula and clavicle. J Bone Joint Surg Am. 2000;82(6):774–80.
9. Hashiguchi H, Ito H. Clinical outcome of the treatment of floating shoulder by osteosynthesis for clavicular fracture alone. J Shoulder Elb Surg. 2003;12(6):589–91.
10. Lin TL, Li YF, Hsu CJ, Hung CH, Lin CC, Fong YC, Hsu HC, Tsai CH. Clinical outcome and radiographic change of ipsilateral scapular neck and clavicular shaft fracture: comparison of operation and conservative treatment. J Orthop Surg Res. 2015;28(10):9–16.
11. Cunningham BP, Bosch L, Swanson D, McLemore R, Rhorer AS, Parikh HR, Albersheim M, Ortega G. The floating flail chest: acute management of an injury combination of the floating shoulder and flail chest. J Orthop Trauma Rehab. 2020;27(1):10–5.
12. Sirmali M, Türüt H, Topçu S, et al. A comprehensive analysis of traumatic rib fractures: morbidity, mortality and management. Eur J Cardiothorac Surg. 2003;24(1):133–8.
13. Lee RB, Bass SM, Morris JA, et al. Three or more rib fractures as an indicator for transfer to a Level I trauma center: a population-based study. J Trauma. 1990;30(6):689–94.
14. Dehghan N, de Mestral C, McKee MD, et al. Flail chest injuries: a review of outcomes and treatment practices from the national trauma data bank. J Trauma Acute Care Surg. 2014;76(2):462–8.
15. Ziegler DW, Agarwal NN. The morbidity and mortality of rib fractures. J Trauma. 1994;37(6):975–9.
16. Ciraulo DL, Elliott D, Mitchell KA, et al. Flail chest as a marker for significant injuries. J Am Coll Surg. 1994;178(5):466–70.
17. Simon B, Ebert J, Bokhari F, et al. Management of pulmonary contusion and flail chest. J Trauma Acute Care Surg. 2012;73(5 Suppl 4):S351–61.
18. Tanaka H, Yukioka T, Yamaguti Y, et al. Surgical stabilization of internal pneumatic stabilization? A prospective randomized study of management of severe flail chest patients. J Trauma. 2002;52(4):727–32. discussion 732
19. Granetzny A, Abd El-Aal M, Emam E, Shalaby A, Boseila A. Surgical versus conservative treatment of flail chest. Evaluation of the pulmonary status. Interact Cardiovasc Thorac Surg. 2005;4(6):583–7.
20. Althausen PL, Shannon S, Watts C, et al. Early surgical stabilization of flail chest with locked plate fixation. J Orthop Trauma. 2011;25(11):641–7.
21. Kilic D, Findikcioglu A, Akin S, et al. Factors affecting morbidity and mortality in flail chest: comparison of anterior and lateral location. Thorac Cardiovasc Surg. 2011;59(01):45–8.
22. Athanassiadi K, Theakos N, Kalantzi N, et al. Prognostic factors in flail-chest patients. Eur J Cardio-Thoracic Surg. 2010;38(4):466–71.
23. Livingston DH, Shogan B, John P, et al. CT diagnosis of rib fractures and the prediction of acute respiratory failure. J Trauma. 2008;64(4):905–11.

24. Cataneo AJ, Cataneo DC, de Oliveira FH, Arruda KA, El Dib R, de Oliveira Carvalho PE. Surgical versus nonsurgical interventions for flail chest. Cochr Database Syst Rev. 2015;2015(7):CD009919.
25. Taylor BC, Fowler TT, French BG, Dominguez N. Clinical outcomes of surgical stabilization of flail chest injury. J Am Acad Orthopaed Surg. 2016;24(8):575–80.
26. Pieracci FM, Majercik S, Ali-Osman F, Ang D, Doben A, Edwards JG, et al. Consensus statement: surgical stabilization of rib fractures rib fracture colloquium clinical practice guidelines. Injury. 2017;48(2):307–21.
27. Chuang CH, Huang CK, Li CY, Hu MH, Lee WPT. Surgical stabilization of the ipsilateral scapula and rib fractures using the mirror Judet approach: a preliminary result. BMC Musculoskelet Disord. 2022;23(105):1–9.

Chapter 11
Special Considerations: Complex Scapular Fractures—Preoperative Planning and Fixation Strategies (Case Based)

Vincenzo Giordano, Robinson Esteves Pires, and Pedro José Labronici

11.1 Case 1

11.1.1 Clinical Setting

A 28-year-old male patient suffered a motorcycle accident and presented a floating shoulder on the left shoulder (non-dominant limb), associated with ipsilateral rib fractures. After clinical and pulmonary stabilization (48 h after the trauma), fracture fixation was performed.

11.1.2 Work-up Images

The 3D CT scan allows for identification of the fracture pattern and preoperative planning (Fig. 11.1).

V. Giordano
Orthopedics Department, Hospital Municipal Miguel Couto, Rio de Janeiro, Brazil

R. E. Pires (✉)
Department of the Locomotor Apparatus, Federal University of Minas Gerais,
Belo Horizonte, Minas Gerais, Brazil

P. J. Labronici
Department of General and Specialized Surgery, Fluminense Federal University,
Niterói, Brazil

© The Author(s), under exclusive license to Springer Nature
Switzerland AG 2024
R. E. Pires et al. (eds.), *Fractures of the Scapula*,
https://doi.org/10.1007/978-3-031-58498-5_11

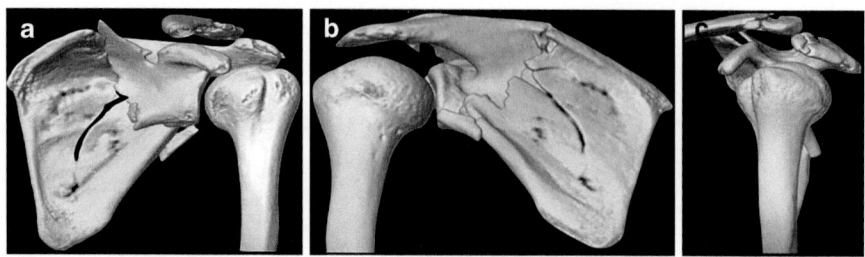

Fig. 11.1 3D reconstruction of the CT scan showing the floating shoulder. (**a**) Anterior view. (**b**) Posterior view. (**c**) Lateral view. Observe the combination of the distal clavicle, scapular neck (with the characteristic triangular avulsion fragment caused by triceps origin) with extension to the scapular body, scapular spine. The patient also presented an asymptomatic os acromiale

11.1.3 Preoperative Planning

11.1.3.1 Patient Positioning

Patient was placed lateral due to the association of the distal clavicle and scapula fractures. Supine positioning to fix the clavicle, followed by prone positioning is also an alternative strategy, with the drawback of surgical extension time, but with the potential advantage of better-quality intraoperative fluoroscopy images.

11.1.3.2 Intraoperative Image

Using the lateral positioning, the C-arm is positioned over the patient. Key intraoperative images include anteroposterior view of the clavicle, Zanca, anteroposterior view of the shoulder, the true anteroposterior view (Grashey view), the axillary view, and the lateral view of the scapula (Y-view).

11.1.3.3 Instruments and Implants

Pointed clamps, small diameter Schanz screws, T-Handle, bone hook, and minidistractor are helpful tools frequently used for fracture reduction. Minifragment 2.4- and 2.7-mm plates and 1/3 tubular plate were the implants used for fracture fixation. However, if available, precontoured clavicle and scapular plates are safe and effective options to be used in this fracture pattern. The hook plate is also an alternative for the clavicle fracture.

11.1.4 Approaches and Fixation Strategy

For the clavicle fracture, a limited longitudinal anterosuperior approach was performed, along the clavicle axis [1]. For the scapula fracture, although several approaches are possible [2–10], including the classic [3] and the modified Judet [2], we decided to use de minimally invasive windows based on the three scapular pillars (scapular spine, medial, and lateral pillars). We started the fixation for the clavicle, followed by the scapular spine and lastly the lateral pillar of the scapula. Our decision was based on the sequence of fixation from the simplest to the most complex fracture. However, we believe that the sequence of fixation, in this case, is up to the surgeon's preference. Fixation was achieved with minifragment 2.4- and 2.7-mm plates, associated with a stronger construct on the lateral pillar, provided by the 1/3 tubular plate (Fig. 11.2). Observe that the avulsion fragment of the triceps was entirely covered by the plate. If necessary, a simple suture passed on the triceps tendon origin is a helpful technique to maintain this fragment in place. It is important to avoid extensive dissections to prevent necrosis of the small triangular fragment.

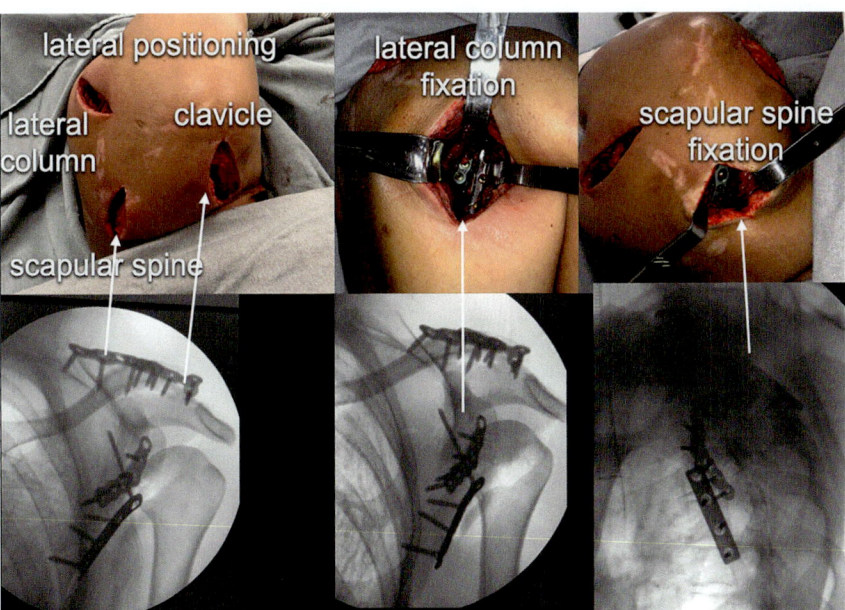

Fig. 11.2 Intraoperative photograph and fluoroscopy images depicting the fixation of the fracture through minimally invasive approach

11.1.4.1 Potential Intraoperative Difficulties

Achieving adequate intraoperative fluoroscopy images using lateral positioning is sometimes challenging, especially in patients with high bone mass index. Reducing the scapular spine prior to the lateral pillar reduction is also demanding due to the muscular forces that act on the fracture site, especially the deltoid muscle. Reducing and fixing the triangular fragment with the avulsed origin of the triceps may be a difficult step of the surgery. Although the previous studies reported that the tenotomy of the triceps can be used to optimize visualization of the inferior glenoid, further studies are necessary to evaluate if leaving this fragment causes a major impact on the functional outcomes. Whenever possible, we prefer to reduce and fix this fragment or suture the triceps origin in one of the plate holes.

11.2 Case 2

11.2.1 Clinical Setting

A 21-year-old male patient suffered a bicycle accident and presented an isolated trauma on the right shoulder (dominant limb). No clinical comorbidities were reported. Absence of neurovascular injuries was documented.

11.2.2 Work-up Images

Radiographic images and CT scan identify an unusual fracture–dislocation of the right shoulder. Observe that the humeral head is posteriorly displaced, and a depression is present at the inferomedial part of the humeral head. The inferior glenoid is displaced anteriorly due to the force of the posteriorly dislocated humeral head. An attempt for reduction of the shoulder at the emergency room was performed, without success. The patient was, therefore, referred to the operating room (Fig. 11.3).

11.2.3 Preoperative Planning

11.2.3.1 Patient Positioning

Patient was placed prone, but lateral oblique positioning is also possible.

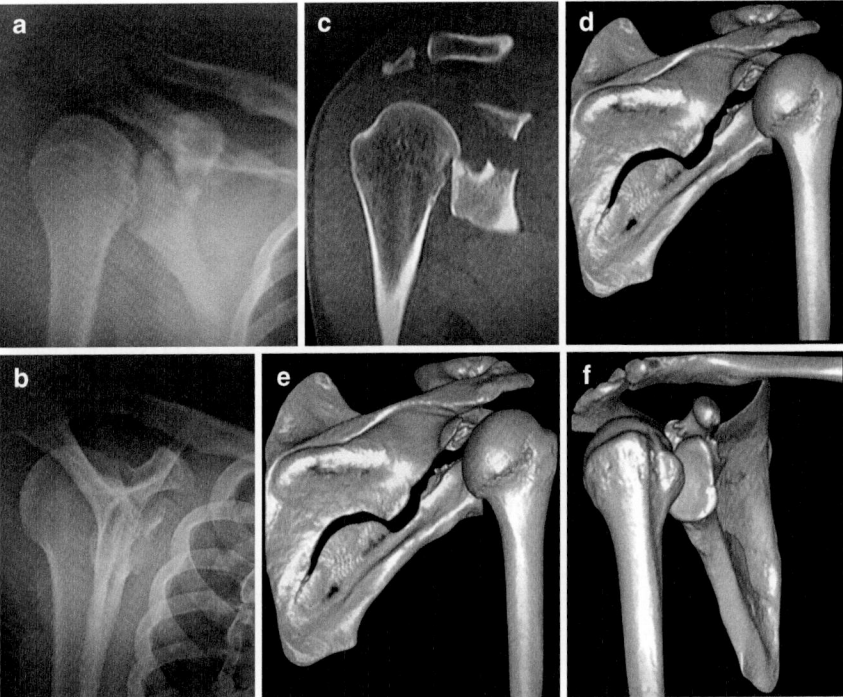

Fig. 11.3 (**a** and **b**) Radiographs of the right shoulder on the anteroposterior and Y views showing the fracture dislocation of the shoulder. (**c**) Coronal cut of the CT scan. Observe the humeral head inferomedially impacted on the glenoid. (**d–f**) 3D reconstruction of the CT scan showing the fracture dislocation. Observe the coracoid process fracture and the anterior displacement of the inferior glenoid, caused by the humeral head

11.2.3.2 Intraoperative Images

Key intraoperative images include the anteroposterior view of the shoulder, the true anteroposterior view (Grashey view), and the lateral view of the scapula (Y-view). Achieving the axillary view with the patient prone is a challenging task.

11.2.3.3 Instruments and Implants

Pointed clamps, small diameter Schanz screws, T-Handle, and bone hook are helpful tools frequently used for this fracture–dislocation reduction. Minifragment 2.7 mm plates were selected for fracture fixation. Nevertheless, precontoured scapular plates and standard or locked 1/3 tubular or 3.5 mm reconstruction plates can also be used for fracture fixation.

11.2.4 Approach and Fixation Strategy

Our preference for this fracture pattern is the modified Judet approach. Using this approach, one can develop the lateral window (between the teres minor and the infraspinatus) and achieve an adequate exposure of the entire lateral pillar of the scapula. Since indirect reduction under shoulder manipulation was not achieved, even after complete exposure of the humeral head, a Hohmann retractor was carefully placed in between the humeral head and the inferior glenoid and slowly moved laterally to allow for the humeral head reduction into the glenoid fossa. Fracture reduction was achieved using pointed reduction clamps, and the fixation was performed with minifragment 2.7 mm locked plates (Fig. 11.4). If a classic or a modified Juded approach is performed, we use a drain for 24 h to prevent a postoperative seroma. When using minimally invasive approaches, the drain is not necessary.

11.2.4.1 Potential Intraoperative Difficulties

Since the humeral head is impacted into the inferior glenoid, achieving reduction of the dislocation is challenging, even using an open direct approach. Although minimally invasive approaches are possible in this case, a limited window can preclude adequate reduction of the fracture–dislocation.

Fixing the coracoid process from the back is demanding, requiring tridimensional understanding of the scapular anatomy.

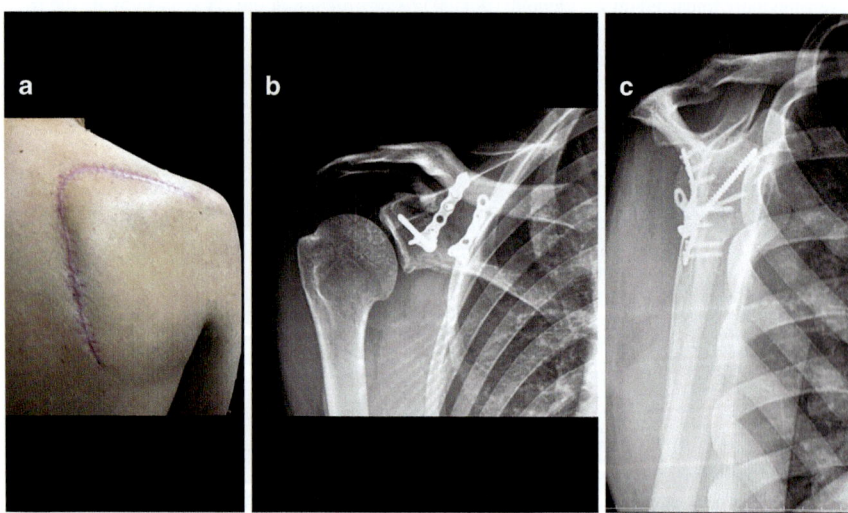

Fig. 11.4 (**a**) Photograph of the posterior aspect of the shoulder after 3 months following the modified Judet approach. (**b** and **c**) Radiographs of the right shoulder in true anteroposterior and lateral (Y) views. Observe anatomic fracture reduction and fixation. Fracture healed uneventfully, and the patient recovered previous functional status

11.3 Case 3

11.3.1 Clinical Setting

A 35-year-old female patient suffered a bicycle accident and presented an isolated trauma on the right shoulder (dominant limb). She also sustained a mild traumatic brain injury, with an initial Glasgow Coma Score of 14 at hospital admission, and a right pneumothorax, which was drained with a chest tube. No clinical comorbidities were reported. Absence of neurovascular injuries was documented.

11.3.2 Work-up Images

Radiographic images and CT scan identify an associated clavicle and glenoid fracture on the right shoulder. Figure 11.5a shows the displaced mid-shaft clavicle fracture and the associated glenoid fracture on the admission X-rays. CT scan (Fig. 11.5b) reveals the shortening of the clavicle fracture, as well as the glenoid fossa involvement. The patient was managed surgically after 48 h of hospital admission.

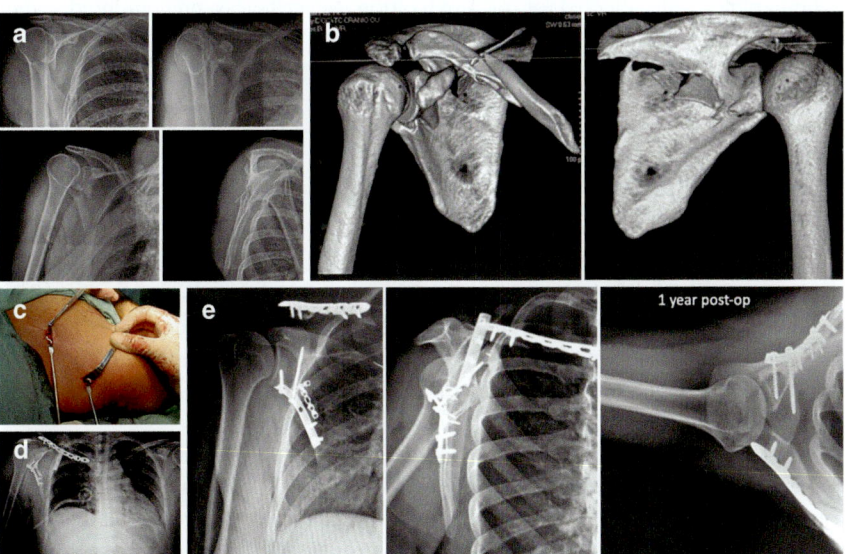

Fig. 11.5 (a) Observe the displaced mid-shaft clavicle fracture and the associated glenoid fracture on the admission X-rays. CT scan (b) reveals shortening of the clavicle fracture, as well as the glenoid fossa involvement. (c) Intraoperative photograph demonstrating the minimally invasive fixation of the clavicle fracture. (d) Immediate postoperative radiograph in anteroposterior view of the chest showing clavicle and scapula fixation with plates and screws. (e) One-year postoperative radiographs showing fracture healing

11.3.3 Preoperative Planning

11.3.3.1 Patient Positioning

Patient was initially placed prone for the management of the scapular fracture, and then repositioned supine in a beach chair position for the clavicle fixation.

11.3.3.2 Intraoperative Images

With the patient prone, intraoperative images include the anteroposterior view of the shoulder, the true anteroposterior view (Grashey view), and the lateral view of the scapula (Y-view). With the patient supine in the beach chair positioning, intraoperative views include the anteroposterior views of the clavicle in neutral, in 30° degrees caudally tilted, and in 30° cranially tilted.

11.3.3.3 Instruments and Implants

Pointed clamps, small diameter Schanz screws, T-Handle, and bone hook are helpful tools frequently used for this fracture–dislocation reduction. Minifragment 2.7 mm plates were selected for fracture fixation. Nevertheless, precontoured scapular plates and standard or locked 1/3 tubular or 3.5 mm reconstruction plates can also be used for fracture fixation.

11.3.4 Approach and Fixation Strategy

For this associated fracture pattern, we used small incision for approaching the medial border of the scapula and the Brodsky approach for the lateral border of the scapula. Using the mini medial approach, the fracture line was adequately exposed and fixed first to reestablish the medial hinge. Then, through the lateral approach, the glenoid fossa and neck were anatomically reduced and fixed. Fracture reduction was achieved and maintained with a 2.7-mm locked plate.

After skin closure and bandages, the patient was repositioned supine, and the clavicle fracture was indirectly reduced and fixed through two small incisions using a precontoured superior clavicle locked plate (Fig. 11.5c). Figure 11.5d shows the immediate postoperative X-ray, demonstrating the satisfactory reduction of both fractures. Figure 11.5e shows the radiographic follow-up after 1 year.

11.3.4.1 Potential Intraoperative Difficulties

Many surgeons prefer to start fixing the clavicle when there is an associated clavicle and scapular fracture. In this particular case, we preferred to start from the scapula to manage the most difficult part of the procedure first to as rapid as we could switch the patient to a supine position. Fixing the mid-shaft clavicle fracture percutaneously is not a complex procedure; however, the surgeon needs to use all intraoperative imaging views to adequately reduce and position the implant. Finally, as stated before, fixing the coracoid process from the back is demanding, requiring tridimensional understanding of the scapular anatomy.

11.4 Case 4

11.4.1 Clinical Setting

A 39-year-old male patient suffered a horse accident, sustaining associated fracture of the right humerus shaft with traumatic radial nerve palsy and an ipsilateral multifragmentary complex scapular fracture. No other skeletal and non-skeletal injuries were observed, and the patient had no clinical comorbidities.

The humerus shaft was managed on emergent basis with open reduction and internal fixation using a lateral large fragment non-locked plate, and radial nerve decompression.

11.4.2 Work-up Images

Radiographic images and CT scan of the right shoulder revealed an Ideberg type VI A associated with a highly comminuted scapula body fracture. Figure 11.6a shows the X-rays and CT images (Fig. 11.6b) of the comminuted scapula fracture. The patient was managed surgically after 7 days of hospital admission.

11.4.3 Preoperative Planning

11.4.3.1 Patient Positioning

Patient was positioned prone with the right arm resting in an arm holder with the elbow flexed at 90°.

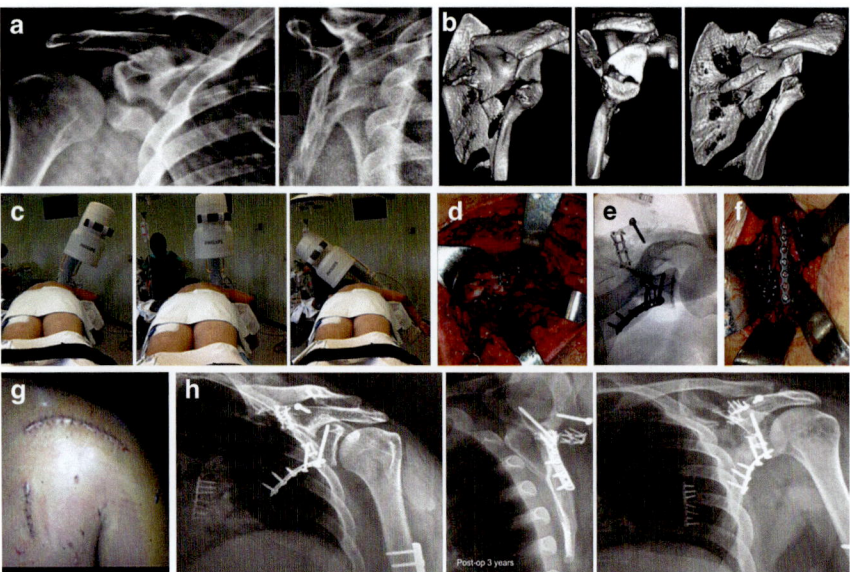

Fig. 11.6 (**a**) Radiographic images and CT scan (**b**) of the right shoulder revealed an Ideberg type VI associated with a highly comminuted scapula body fracture. (**c**) Observe the C-arm positioning with the patient prone. (**d**) A limited Van Noort approach was performed to reduce both the spine of the scapula and the glenoid fossa component. (**e**) Observe the 2.4-mm plate associated with a 3.5-mm screw and washer in a lag screw technique were used to fix the spine of the scapula. The Obremskey and Liman interval was dissected to expose the glenoid fossa fracture. The glenoid fossa was reduced and maintained with a 2.4-mm plate. Final fixation was performed using a 3.5-mm one-third tubular plate in the lateral border of the scapula acting as a buttressing plate. (**f**) A small 2.4-mm straight plate was used to fix the medial border. (**g**) Observe the aspect of the surgical wounds. (**h**) Radiographic follow-up after 3 years showing fracture healing

11.4.3.2 Intraoperative Images

With the patient prone, intraoperative images include the anteroposterior view of the shoulder, the true anteroposterior view (Grashey view), and the lateral view of the scapula (Y-view). Observe the C-arm positioning with the patient prone (Fig. 11.6c).

11.4.3.3 Instruments and Implants

Pointed clamps, small diameter Schanz screws, T-Handle, and bone hook are helpful tools frequently used for this fracture–dislocation reduction. Minifragment 2.4- and 2.7-mm plates were selected for fracture fixation. Nevertheless, precontoured scapular plates and standard or locked 1/3 tubular or 3.5 mm reconstruction plates can also be used for fracture fixation.

11.4.3.4 Approach and Fixation Strategy

A limited Van Noort approach was performed to reduce both the spine of the scapula and the glenoid fossa component. A 2.4-mm plate associated with a 3.5-mm screw and washer in a lag screw technique were used to fix the spine of the scapula (Fig. 11.6d). Then, the Obremskey and Liman interval was dissected to expose the glenoid fossa fracture. The glenoid fossa was reduced and maintained with a 2.4-mm plate. Final fixation was performed using a 3.5-mm one-third tubular plate in the lateral border of the scapula acting as a buttressing plate (Fig. 11.6e). Finally, a small incision for approaching the medial border of the scapula was done to adequately expose the medial fracture line and reestablish the medial hinge. A small 2.4-mm straight plate was used to fix the medial border (Fig. 11.6f). Figure 11.6g shows the aspect of the surgical wounds. Figure 11.6h shows the radiographic follow-up after 3 years. The patient regained full range of motion and returned to his pre-injury level of activity.

11.4.3.5 Potential Intraoperative Difficulties

The use of the Van Noort approach is adequate to approach both the scapula spine and the glenoid neck and fossa. Surgeons need to develop the Obremskey and Liman interval and take care to not damage the suprascapular nerve, denervating the infraspinatus muscle. Fixing the medial border of the scapula fracture reestablishes the medial hinge, thus adding stability to the lateral fixation.

11.5 Case 5

11.5.1 Clinical Setting

A 33-year-old male patient suffered a motorcycle accident, sustaining a right multi-fragmentary complex scapular fracture. No other skeletal and non-skeletal injuries were observed, neurovascular was intact, and the patient had no clinical comorbidities.

11.5.2 Work-up Images

Radiographic images and CT scan of the right shoulder revealed an Ideberg type VI A associated with a coracoid base scapula body fracture. Figure 11.7a, b show the X-rays and CT images of the comminuted scapula fracture. The patient was managed surgically after 5 days of hospital admission.

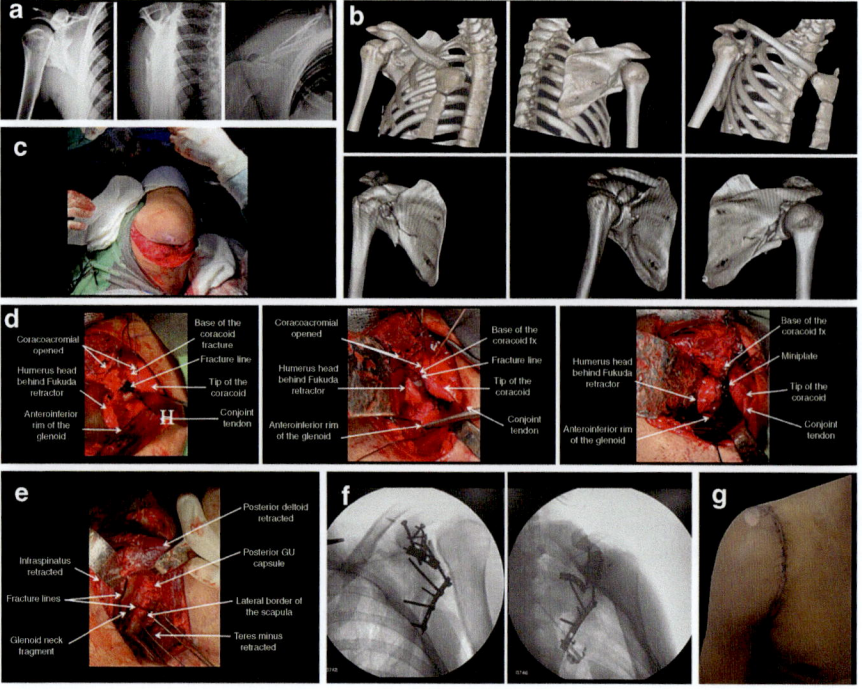

Fig. 11.7 (**a** and **b**) Radiographs and 3D CT scan showing a complex scapular fracture. (**c**) Intraoperative photograph showing the extended saber approach. (**d** and **e**) Intraoperative photographs showing the anterior (**d**) and posterior (**e**) aspects of the extended saber approach. (**f**) Fluoroscopy images showing fracture reduction and fixation. (**g**) Clinical aspect of the wound

11.5.3 Preoperative Planning

11.5.3.1 Patient Positioning

Patient was positioned in a floppy lateral position with the right arm prepped and draped.

11.5.3.2 Intraoperative Images

With the patient prone, intraoperative images include the anteroposterior view of the shoulder, the true anteroposterior view (Grashey view), the lateral view of the scapula (Y-view), the axillary view, and the Stryker let view.

11.5.3.3 Instruments and Implants

Pointed clamps, small diameter Schanz screws, T-Handle, and bone hook are helpful tools frequently used for this fracture–dislocation reduction. Minifragment 2.0-mm plates and 3.5-mm small fragment plates were selected for fracture fixation.

11.5.4 Approach and Fixation Strategy

An extended saber approach following posterior in line with the Brodsky approach was performed to reduce both the coracoid process of the scapula and the glenoid fossa and neck components (Fig. 11.7c). The anterior window was developed first. Due to the integrity of both the coracoclavicular and coracoacromial ligaments, the fracture of the base of the coracoid was inaccessible. Thus, we need to open the coracoacromial ligament to expose the coracoid fracture line and reduce it. A 2.0-mm plate associated with a 3.5-mm screw and washer in a lag screw technique were used to fix the coracoid process of the scapula (Fig. 11.7d). After the fixation was done, the coracoacromial ligament was repaired. Then, the posterior window was developed, and the Obremskey and Liman interval was dissected to expose the glenoid fossa fracture (Fig. 11.7e). The glenoid fossa was reduced and maintained with a 2.0-mm plate. Final fixation was performed using a 3.5-mm one-third tubular plate in the lateral border of the scapula acting as a buttressing plate (Fig. 11.7f). Figure 11.7g shows the wound aspect after fracture fixation. Figure 11.8 shows fracture reduction and fixation. The patient regained full range of motion and returned to his pre-injury level of activity.

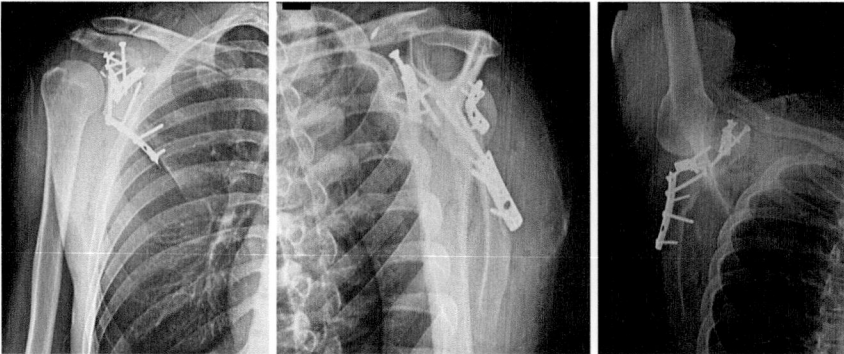

Fig. 11.8 Postoperative radiographs showing adequate fracture reduction and fixation

11.5.4.1 Potential Intraoperative Difficulties

The use of the extended saber approach is a rare indication, but it seems adequate to simultaneously approach fractures of the base of the coracoid process and of the neck and glenoid fossa simultaneously. The use of two distinct approaches could be done, still in a floppy lateral position. The opening of the coracoacromial ligament was necessary since there was no space to approach the fracture of the base of the coracoid process, but it needs to be repaired. Finally, surgeons need to develop the Obremskey and Liman gap and take care not to injure the suprascapular nerve by denervating the infraspinatus muscle.

11.6 Case 6

11.6.1 Clinical Setting

A 40-year-old male patient suffered a motorcycle accident, sustaining a right multifragmentary scapular fracture associated with a floating thorax with bilateral hemothorax. Bilateral chest tube was done to drain the hemothorax. No other skeletal and non-skeletal injuries were observed, neurovascular was intact, and the patient had no clinical comorbidities.

11.6.2 Work-up Images

Radiographic images and CT scan of the right shoulder revealed an Ideberg type VI A associated with a multifragmentary scapular body fracture. Figure 11.9 shows the X-rays (a) and CT (b) images of the comminuted scapula fracture. The patient was managed surgically after 3 days of hospital admission.

11.6.3 Preoperative Planning

11.6.3.1 Patient Positioning

Patient was positioned lateral with the right arm prepped and draped.

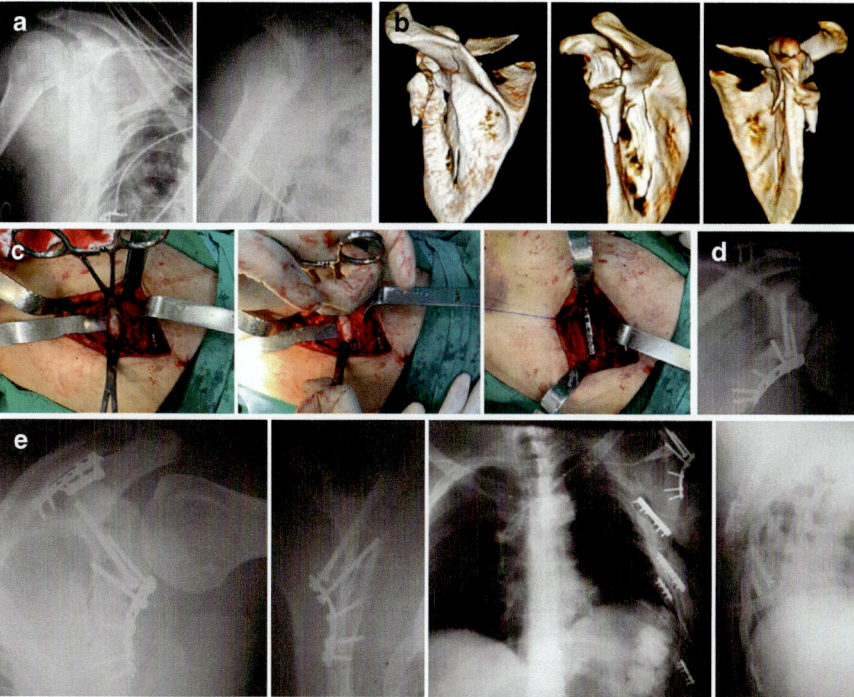

Fig. 11.9 (**a** and **b**) Radiographs and CT scan showing a complex fracture of the scapula associated with multiple rib fractures. (**c**) Intraoperative photographs showing rob reduction and fixation with plates and screws. (**d** and **e**) Postoperative radiographs showing the scapular fracture reduction and fixation, as well as the ribs fixation

11.6.3.2 Intraoperative Images

Intraoperative images include the anteroposterior view of the shoulder, the true anteroposterior view (Grashey view), the lateral view of the scapula (Y-view), and the axillary view.

11.6.3.3 Instruments and Implants

Pointed clamps, small diameter Schanz screws, T-Handle, and bone hook are helpful tools frequently used for this fracture–dislocation reduction. Minifragment 2.0-mm plates and 3.5-mm small fragment plates were selected for fracture fixation.

11.6.4 Approach and Fixation Strategy

A posterior Brodsky approach was performed to reduce both the scapula spine and the glenoid fossa and neck components. The scapula spine was reduced and fixed using two orthogonal 2.0-mm plates. Then, the Obremskey and Liman interval was dissected to expose the glenoid fossa fracture. The glenoid fossa was reduced and fixed using a 3.5-mm one-third tubular plate in the lateral border of the scapula acting as a buttressing plate. Finally, a 4.5-mm cortical screw was used from posterior to anterior to fix the coracoid process in a lag screw technique.

A second approach using an oblique incision at the level of the scapular angle was performed to expose both the scapular angle and the fractured ribs (Fig. 11.9c). A 2.0-mm plate was used to fix the scapular angle. Then, the sixth, seventh, and ninth costal arches were reduced and fixed using 2.0-mm plates (Fig. 11.9d, e). The patient was discharged 10 days after the surgical procedure. He returned for 2 outpatient visits and then he was lost to follow-up.

11.6.4.1 Potential Intraoperative Difficulties

Fractures of the ipsilateral scapula are common in patients undergoing surgical stabilization of subscapular rib fractures [11]. However, there are no current decision algorithms that define the benefits or when to surgically stabilize rib fractures in this setting [11, 12]. All treatment modalities, fixing subscapular rib fractures or not, seem feasible [12]. Although the added value of rib and scapula fixation has yet to be proven in large multicenter studies, we feel that with fixation of both fractures, there is an improvement in lung function as well as pain, which allows for earlier initiation of the mechanical and respiratory physiotherapy protocol.

References

1. Pires RE, Giordano V, Mendes de Souza FS, Labronici PJ. Current challenges and controversies in the management of scapular fractures: a review. Patient Saf Surg. 2021;15(6):1–18.
2. Judet R. Traitement chirurgical des fractures de l'omoplate. Acta Orthop Belg. 1964;30:673–8.
3. Obremskey WT, Lyman JR. A modified Judet approach to the scapula. J Orthop Trauma. 2004;18(10):696–9.
4. Ebraheim NA, Mekhail AO, Padanilum TG, Yeasting RA. Anatomic considerations for a modified posterior approach to the scapula. Clin Orthop. 1997;334:136–43.
5. Wijdicks CA, Armitage BM, Anavian J, Schroder LK, Cole PA. Vulnerable neurovasculature with a posterior approach to the scapula. Clin Orthop. 2009;467(8):2011–7.
6. Harmer LS, Phelps KD, Crickard CV, Sample KM, Andrews EB, Hamid N, et al. A comparison of exposure between the classic and modified Judet approaches to the scapula. J Orthop Trauma. 2016;30(5):235–9.
7. Salassa TE, Hill BW, Cole PA. Quantitative comparison of exposure for the posterior Judet approach to the scapula with and without deltoid takedown. J Shoulder Elb Surg. 2014;23(11):1747–52.

8. Garlich JM, Samuel K, Nelson TJ, Monfiston C, Kremen T, Metzger MF, et al. Infraspinatus tenotomy improves glenoid visualization with the modified Judet approach. J Orthop Trauma. 2020;34(3):158–62.
9. Gauger EM, Cole PA. Surgical technique: a minimally invasive approach to scapula neck and body fractures. Clin Orthop. 2011;469(12):3390–9.
10. Jiang B, Lu J, Kang X, Li L, Jiang S, Gong X. Minimally invasive surgery for complex scapular fractures through small incisions combined with titanium miniplate fixation. Int J Clin Exp Med. 2016;9(9):18124–32.
11. Gargur Assuncao A, Leasia K, White T, Majercik S, Gardner S, Mauffrey C, Parry J, Moore EE, Pieracci FM. Characterization and influence of ipsilateral scapula fractures among patients who undergo surgical stabilization of sub-scapular rib fractures. Eur J Orthop Surg Traumatol. 2021;31(3):429–34.
12. Veelen N, Houwert RM, Babst R, Link BC, van de Wall BJM. Treatment and outcome in combined scapula and rib fractures: a retrospective study. Eur J Orthop Surg Traumatol. 2023;33(6):2337–45.

Chapter 12
Periprosthetic Scapular Fractures Following Reverse Shoulder Arthroplasty

Robinson Esteves Pires, Parag Shah, Chittaranjan Patel, and Vincenzo Giordano

12.1 Epidemiology and Risk Factors

Reverse shoulder arthroplasty procedures presented a dramatic growth in the last decade. However, an occasional complication has drawn attention, especially for shoulder and arthroplasty surgeons, the scapular spine or acromial fracture following RSA.

The periprosthetic scapular fracture occurs more frequently at the base of the acromion or close to the spinoglenoid junction [1]. This rare complication may occur intraoperatively, just a few weeks or several months after the surgical procedure, with a peak of 9 months and an incidence of up to 4.3%, depending on the specific prosthesis design [1–4].

One of the earliest published series on this complication was published in 2013. The authors found an incidence of 10.2% of acromial stress fractures in lateralized glenoids [5]. Lateralized glenosphere seems to be more associated with periprosthetic scapular fractures than medialized. Rate of postoperative scapular fractures with BIO-RSA at 16.7% was also significantly higher than standard reverse shoulder arthroplasty at 9.1% [6]. The overall rate of scapular and acromial fractures for

R. E. Pires (✉)
Department of the Locomotor Apparatus, Federal University of Minas Gerais, Belo Horizonte, Minas Gerais, Brazil

P. Shah
Department of Orthopaedics, KD Hospital, Ahmedabad, Gujarat, India

C. Patel
Nirali Hospital, Navsari, Gujarat, India

V. Giordano
Orthopedics Department, Hospital Municipal Miguel Couto, Rio de Janeiro, Brazil

© The Author(s), under exclusive license to Springer Nature Switzerland AG 2024
R. E. Pires et al. (eds.), *Fractures of the Scapula*,
https://doi.org/10.1007/978-3-031-58498-5_12

all designs was 2.8% [1]. Biomechanical data showed that glenosphere lateralization of 10 mm increases stress placed on the acromion during functional shoulder activities by approximately 17% [7].

The comparison of surgical approaches, including the classic deltopectoral, anterosuperior, and superolateral, has not shown any association with increased risk of periprosthetic scapular fracture [8–10]. Although the current literature on whether deltoid lengthening or shortening is related to periprosthetic scapular fractures remains controversial [1, 8], Zmistowski et al. [3] identified decreased deltoid lengthening as an independent predictor of acromial fracture. A shortened deltoid theoretically exerts an important force on the acromion during shoulder motion [3].

The presence of an intact rotator cuff, particularly the subscapularis tendon, also has been identified to increase the risk of acromial and scapular spine fractures after RSA. Giles et al. [8], in a biomechanical study, showed that an intact rotator cuff acts as a deltoid antagonist, thereby increasing the work load of the deltoid, consequently increasing the acromial stress. An intact subscapularis may lead to increased posterior erosion and may involve the scapular spine [11].

A potential risk factor may be related to the site of emergence of screws used to fix the glenosphere. Therefore, it is recommended the use of shorter screws aimed at the base of the coracoid for baseplate fixation [1]. Ascione et al. [4] reported that more than 50% of acromial fractures following RSA occurred at the distal tip of the superior screw, which is consistent with the theory that a superior screw engaging the scapular spine acts as a stress riser, thereby increasing the risk of a periprosthetic scapular fracture. Another biomechanical study showed that metaglene fixation incorporating a screw superior to its central axis presents a lower load-to-failure than RSA constructs with only an inferior screw placed inferiorly the central glenoid axis [9]. The authors reported that after changing their surgical technique to an "inferior-only" metaglene fixation technique, the incidence of fracture following RSA dropped from 4.4% to 0% [9]. However, it is noteworthy that the implant used in this study allows for placement of three inferior locking screws, whereas several other implants allow for just a single inferior locking screw placement. Fixation of metaglene construct with just a single inferior screw may be insufficient to prevent implant instability [10]. Mayne et al. [12] recommend the use of a short posterior screw ($\leq$20 mm) for metaglene fixation to prevent placing into the scapular spine.

Onlay humeral stem is one of the innovations of RSA. However, in a case series of 1953 RSA using Grammont-style prosthesis, Neyton et al. [13] reported that the incidence of scapular fractures in the inlay humeral group was 1.3%, compared to 4.3% in the onlay group. Larose et al. [14] also concluded in a systemic review that onlay humeral tray design has a higher rate of scapular spine fracture. The increased distalization that happens with an onlay stem may be associated with a higher incidence of scapular spine fractures. Taylor et al. [15] reported that the transection of the coracoacromial ligament significantly altered the stress on the acromion and scapular spine by up to 19%. The authors recommend preservation of the coracoacromial ligament during surgical exposure for RSA, to decrease the risk of scapular spine fractures.

The majority of periprosthetic scapular fractures are atraumatic, being considered an insufficiency fracture associated with low bone mineral density [5]. A previous history of shoulder surgery, including rotator cuff repair and acromioplasty, is frequently associated (Fig. 12.1).

The risk of intraoperative periprosthetic scapular fracture deserves attention, particularly in patients with rheumatoid arthritis, osteopenia, and in the revision procedure setting [10].

Tenderness or pain at the scapular spine or base of the acromion may be present, even in the absence of a radiologically proven fracture. These findings usually occur with a peak at 7.3 months after RSA [10]. King et al. [16], in a systematic review of the literature, reported that periprosthetic scapular fractures occurred most frequently following the arthroplasty procedure for inflammatory arthritis (10.8%), and less frequently for post-traumatic arthritis (2.1%) and acute humeral or glenoid fracture (0%).

Periprosthetic scapular fractures are the second most common complication following RSA, responding for approximately 20% of all complications, being behind only of the prosthesis instability [10].

Compared to fractures following anatomic total shoulder arthroplasty, periprosthetic fractures following RSA occur more than three times as frequently [10].

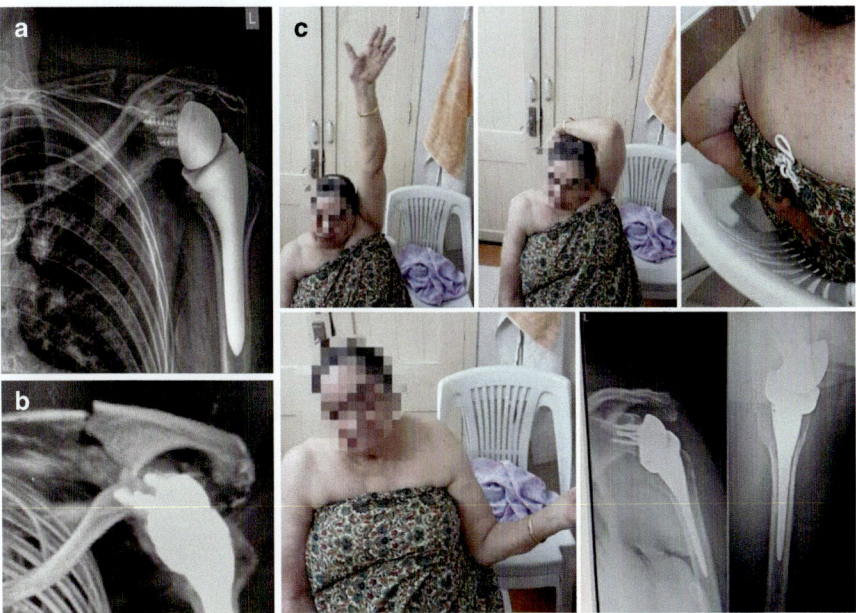

Fig. 12.1 (**a** and **b**) represent an 85-year-old lady, with an atraumatic fracture of the scapular spine 5 months after the index surgery, leading to acute pain and loss of function. (**c**): An asymptomatic acromion fracture detected incidentally at 6 year follow-up after a reverse shoulder arthroplasty. Patient continued to be painless and functional

12.2 Treatment

Treatment of scapular spine and acromial fractures following reverse shoulder arthroplasty remains challenging, and the outcomes, regardless the treatment method, are still unpredictable (Fig. 12.2). The functional outcomes of the reverse arthroplasty procedure are obviously worse in those patients who suffer a periprosthetic scapular fracture, especially in those with attempted nonoperative management in an abduction brace [1].

If symptoms of stress reaction are present, an abduction brace for around 6 weeks is recommended, until complete relief of the clinical scenario (Fig. 12.3).

The Levy et al. [5] classification system is based on the origin of the deltoid. This anatomic classification is universally used to guide the treatment (Fig. 12.4). Nonoperative management is recommended for nondisplaced fractures affecting the acromion and the segment of spine suspending the acromion (classified as types I and II by Levy et al. [5]) [17, 18]. Nonoperative treatment consists of immobilization using an abduction brace also for 6 weeks, followed by gradual increase shoulder motion [10].

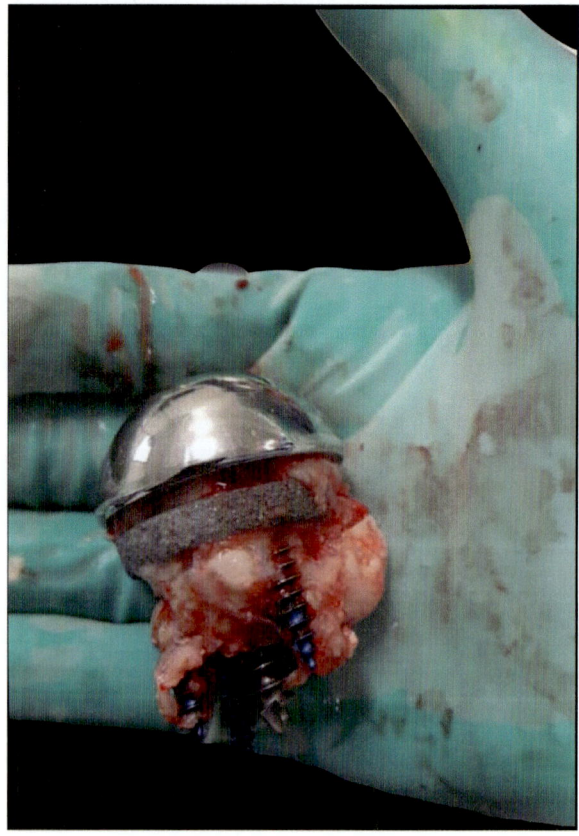

Fig. 12.2 An acute, but trivial trauma 8 weeks after RSA for cuff tear arthroplasty. Patient presented with dislocation and a fracture of the vault leading to an "amputation" of the glenoid

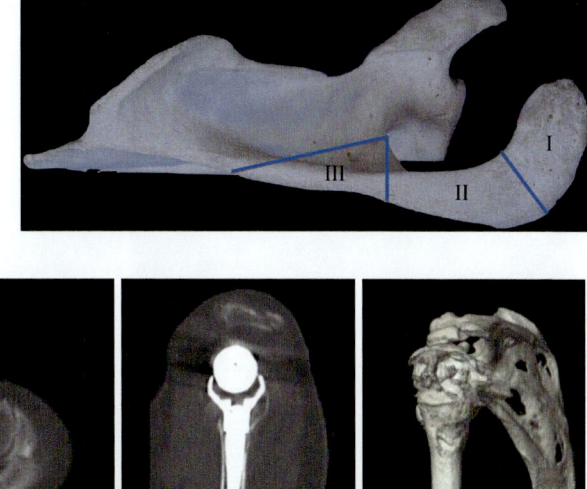

Fig. 12.3 Illustration of the Levy et al. [5] classification system for periprosthetic scapular fractures following RSA

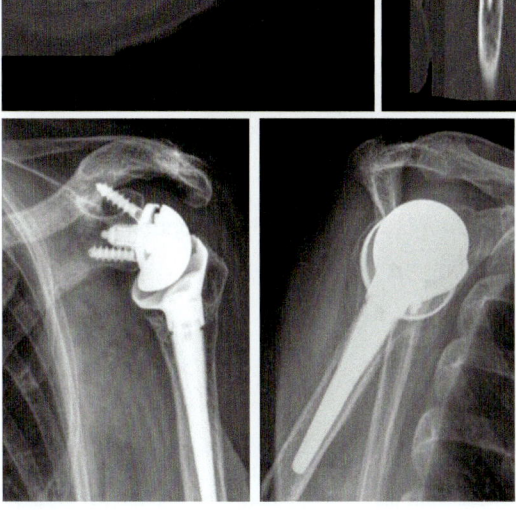

Fig. 12.4 A 77-year-old female patient presented a proximal humeral fracture with severe displacement. A reverse shoulder arthroplasty was performed. The patient evolved with a late periprosthetic acromial fracture that was managed nonoperatively. (Courtesy: Dr Jaime Guiotti Filho, Chief of the Shoulder and Elbow Service, Orthopaedic Institute of Goiania (Brazil))

Operative management is recommended for displaced fractures. Levy type 3 fractures are more at risk of nonunion, whereas a greater amount of the deltoid is attached distal to the fracture level, thereby increasing the risk of a secondary displacement. Tension band wiring and plate fixation are the most used treatment methods to fix these fracture patterns (Fig. 12.5). Depending on the bone and fragments sizes, as well as the amount of force acting over the distal fragment, 3.5 mm

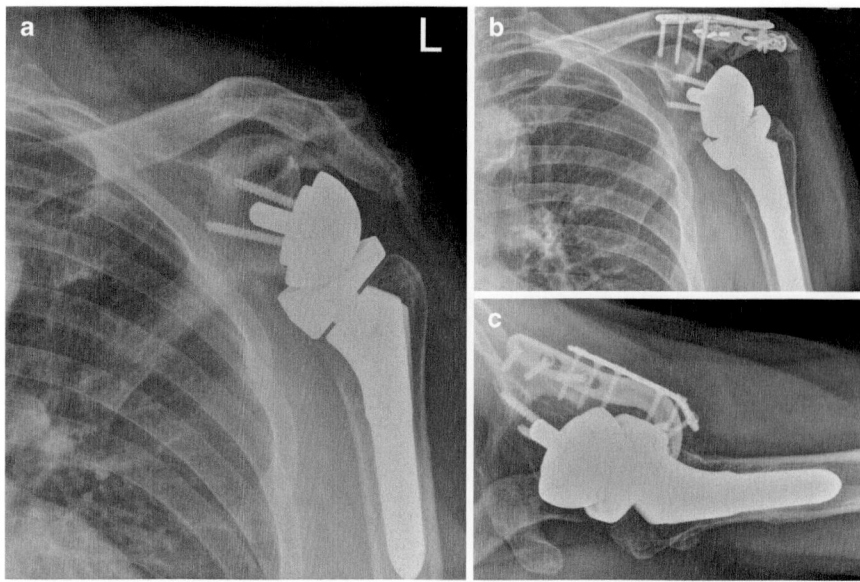

Fig. 12.5 Operative management for a persistently symptomatic fracture of the scapular spine treated with dual pre-contoured plates. (**a**) Preoperative radiograph showing the periprosthetic scapular spine fracture. (**b** and **c**) Postoperative images showing fracture fixation with double plating. (Case courtesy Mr. Amol Tambe, Consultant Shoulder and Upper Limb Surgeon, UK)

reconstruction locking plate or minifragment 2.4 or 2.7 mm plates can be safely used. Revision of reverse shoulder arthroplasty may be another option, particularly on the presence of fixation failure or prosthesis instability.

References

1. Limb D. Scapula fractures: a review. EFORT Open Rev. 2021;6:518–25.
2. Teusink MJ, Otto RJ, Cottrell BJ, Frankle MA. What is the effect of postoperative scapular fracture on outcomes of reverse shoulder arthroplasty? J Shoulder Elb Surg. 2014;23:782–90.
3. Zmistowski B, Gutman M, Horvath Y, Abboud JA, Williams GR Jr, Namdari S. Acromial stress fracture following reverse total shoulder arthroplasty: incidence and predictors. J Shoulder Elb Surg. 2020;29:799–806.
4. Ascione F, Kilian CM, Laughlin MS, et al. Increased scapular spine fractures after reverse shoulder arthroplasty with a humeral onlay short stem: an analysis of 485 consecutive cases. J Shoulder Elb Surg. 2018;27:2183–90.
5. Levy JC, Anderson C, Samson A. Classification of postoperative acromial fractures following reverse shoulder arthroplasty. J Bone Joint Surg Am. 2013;95(e104):1–7.
6. Kirzner N, Paul E, Moaveni A. Reverse shoulder arthroplasty vs BIO-RSA: clinical and radiographic outcomes at short term follow up. J Orthop Surg Res. 2018;13:256.
7. Wong MT, Langohr GDG, Athwal GS, Johnson JA. Implant positioning in reverse shoulder arthroplasty has an impact on acromial stresses. J Shoulder Elb Surg. 2016;25:1889–95.

8. Giles JW, Langohr GDG, Johnson JA, Athwal GS. The rotator cuff muscles are antagonists after reverse total shoulder arthroplasty. J Shoulder Elb Surg. 2016;25:1592–600.
9. Kennon JC, Lu C, McGee-Lawrence ME, Crosby LA. Scapula fracture incidence in reverse total shoulder arthroplasty using screws above or below metaglene central cage: clinical and biomechanical outcomes. J Shoulder Elb Surg. 2017;26:1023–30.
10. Brusalis CM, Taylor SA. Periprosthetic fractures in reverse Total shoulder arthroplasty: current concepts and advances in management. Curr Rev Musculoskelet Med. 2020;13:509–19.
11. Farshad M, Gerber C. Reverse total shoulder arthroplasty-from the most to the least common complication. Int Orthop. 2010;34(8):1075–82. [published correction in Int Orthop. 2011;35(3):455].
12. Mayne IP, Bell SN, Wright W, Coghlan JA. Acromial and scapular spine fractures after reverse total shoulder arthroplasty. Shoulder Elbow. 2016;8:90–100.
13. Neyton L, Erickson J, Ascione F, Bugelli G, Lunini E, Walch G. Grammont Award 2018: scapular fractures in reverse shoulder arthroplasty (Grammont style): prevalence, functional, and radiographic results with minimum 5-year follow-up. J Shoulder Elb Surg. 2019;28:260–7.
14. Larose G, Fisher ND, Gambhir N, Alben MG, Zuckerman JD, Virk MS, Kwon YW. Inlay verses onlay humeral design for reverse shoulder arthrpoplasty: a systemic review and meta-analysis. J Shoulder Elb Surg. 2022;31(11):2410–20.
15. Taylor SA, Shah S, Chen X, Gentile J, Gulotta LV, Dines JS, Dines DD, Cordasco FA, Warren RF, Kontaxis A. Scapular ring preservation: coracoacromial ligament transection increases scapular spine strains following reverse total shoulder arthroplasty. J Bone Joint Surg Am. 2020;102(15):1358–64.
16. King JJ, Dalton SS, Gulotta LV, Wright TW, Schoch BS. How common are acromial and scapular spine fractures after reverse shoulder arthroplasty? A systematic review. Bone Joint J. 2019;101-B:627–34.
17. Cho CH, Rhee YG, Yoo JC, et al. Incidence and risk factors of acromial fracture following reverse total shoulder arthroplasty. J Shoulder Elb Surg. 2021;30:57–64.
18. Bohsali KI, Bois AJ, Wirth MA. Complications of shoulder arthroplasty. J Bone Joint Surg Am. 2017;99:256–69.

Chapter 13
Rehabilitation After Scapular Fractures

Andrea Lopes Sauers, Rita Ator, and Jaime González

13.1 Introduction

Scapular fractures are rare, comprising only 1% of all fractures and 5% of all shoulder fractures [1]. Typically, they result from high-impact trauma, including motor vehicle accidents and falls, and may be accompanied by multi-system injuries [2–4]. Most scapular fractures are not displaced or are minimally displaced and are amenable to conservative, nonsurgical treatment using short-term immobilization and mobility exercises to prevent frozen shoulder [1, 2, 5].

Fractures with significant displacement can cause long-term morbidity and poor functional outcomes. Thus, open reduction and internal fixation may be recommended to reduce pain and disability [1, 5]. Recent attention has been given to managing scapular fractures following reverse shoulder arthroplasty (RSA) [5, 6]. These periprosthetic fractures, including stress and frank fractures, are typically atraumatic, from low-energy mechanisms, and may require surgical treatment [5].

There is a paucity of literature on the rehabilitation of scapular fractures. Since they are rare, only case series and case reports are available [3, 4]. Therefore, the purpose of this chapter is to summarize current concepts and to provide recommendations for the rehabilitation of patients following scapular fractures to aid in decision-making.

A. Lopes Sauers (✉) · R. Ator
Physical Therapy Program – College of Health Sciences, Midwestern University, Glendale, AZ, USA

J. González
Physical Therapy Program – College of Health Professions, University of Texas Rio Grande Valley, Edinburg, TX, USA

© The Author(s), under exclusive license to Springer Nature Switzerland AG 2024
R. E. Pires et al. (eds.), *Fractures of the Scapula*, https://doi.org/10.1007/978-3-031-58498-5_13

13.2 Physical Therapy Evaluation

Given that scapular fractures typically occur in association with other traumatic injuries, an interprofessional team operating within a collaborative practice model is ideal. Effective communication between interprofessional team members is critical throughout the rehabilitation process [1]. Once the patient is referred to physical therapy after scapular fracture, the physical therapist conducts an evaluation to determine short- and long-term goals. The history and examination findings should guide the evaluation and intervention focus [7]. The primary scapular fracture treatment (non-operative versus surgical fixation), healing phase, and presence of comorbidities or associated injuries (i.e., nerve or muscle injuries, rib fracture, presence of "floating shoulder") should be considered when selecting tests and measures. These tests and measures should be valid and reliable and may include (1) shoulder range of motion (ROM) measured with a universal goniometer or a digital inclinometer; (2) shoulder strength measured with a handheld dynamometer; (3) patient-reported outcome measures (PROs) [8].

A three-staged approach for rehabilitation classification for shoulder disorders, the *Staged Algorithm for Rehabilitation Classification* (STAR-Shoulder), has been described and validated to assess and guide the rehabilitation progress by the level of irritability and identified impairments [7, 9] (Table 13.1) and may be used to evaluate patients after scapular fractures. A clinical practice guideline for shoulder pain and mobility deficits recommends that physical therapists rate tissue irritability to guide the intensity of rehabilitation intervention [10]. Tissue irritability frameworks have been popular among physical therapists whose clinical practice is heavily grounded in manual therapy [11–15]. The STAR-Shoulder has been demonstrated to be a valid and reliable classification system for symptom irritability [9].

The STAR-Shoulder stages are categorized as low, moderate, and high irritability and use pain levels, the relationship between pain and motion (active and passive ROM), and self-reported disability for rating [7, 9] (Table 13.1). The original

Table 13.1 Shoulder tissue irritability classification

High irritability	Moderate irritability	Low irritability
High pain ($\geq$7/10)	Moderate pain (4–6/10)	Low pain ($\leq$3/10)
Consistent night or resting pain	Intermittent night or resting pain	Absent night or resting pain
AROM < PROM	AROM ~ PROM	AROM = PROM
High disability	Moderate disability	Low disability
Pain before end of ROM	Pain at the end of ROM	Minimal pain with overpressure

Reprinted from SM Kareha, PW McClure, A Fernandez-Fernandez, Reliability and concurrent validity of shoulder tissue irritability classification. Phys Ther. 2021;101(3):1–8 with permission from Oxford University Press on behalf of the American Physical Therapy Association
AROM active range of motion, *PROM* passive range of motion, *ROM* range of motion

STAR-Shoulder validation study [9] assessed self-reported levels of pain and disability using three different PROs: the FOTO Shoulder Computerized Adaptive Test (SCAT) [16], the Penn Shoulder Score (PSS) [17], and the American Shoulder and Elbow Surgeons Score (ASES) [18]. These 3 PROs have been widely used, and their validity and reliability have been tested across populations with different shoulder disorders [9, 19]. The physical therapist may consider these PROs when using the STAR-Shoulder approach to guide decision-making for intervention strategies in patients after scapular fractures. The stage of irritability can be directly matched to the physical intensity of the intervention [7, 9]. Regular testing and monitoring throughout rehabilitation should be done to define the irritability stage and intensity of intervention [7, 9, 14].

In addition to the tests and measures mentioned above, the physical therapist should consider performing a clinical assessment of scapulothoracic dysfunction. The scapular fracture as the primary source of injury may contribute to short-term and long-term scapulothoracic and shoulder muscle imbalance and scapular dyskinesis associated with shoulder symptoms. A recommendation for assessing scapular dyskinesis is using the *scapular dyskinesis test* [20–22]. Symptom alteration tests including the *scapular assistance test* [23] and the *scapular reposition test* [24] may be performed to decide if the scapular dyskinesis contributes to the patient's symptoms [25].

13.3 Rehabilitation After Conservative Management Following Scapular Fracture

Conservative management of scapular fracture can range from watchful waiting to a more active approach, focusing on the areas of deficit and healing. Conservative or nonsurgical management may be recommended in noncomplex simple to moderate scapular fractures with no or minimal displacement and includes stabilization with a sling for the first 2–3 weeks guided by pain [2]. Once the pain has subsided, progressive full passive and active-assisted ROM is indicated. The STAR-Shoulder classification based on tissue irritability and identified physical impairments can be helpful to guide the intensity of physical stress of rehabilitation intervention after nonsurgical management of scapular fracture [7, 9] (Table 13.1). This classification may complement the primary pathoanatomical diagnosis of scapular fracture to correct the impairments caused by the injury that may lead to additional physical stress to the scapula and surrounding tissue. Using this rating system, the physical therapist may develop a specific treatment plan that is modifiable as the patient moves through the episode of care. Activity modification and ROM restoration must precede high-demand functional restoration [9]. Fracture healing time should also be considered, especially in the early phases of rehabilitation following scapular fracture.

In order to achieve effective motion, stability, and control of the forces exerted at the shoulder and scapulothoracic joints, adequate scapular muscle balance is integral. The modified algorithm for scapular rehabilitation may be used when scapulothoracic muscle dysfunction is present (Fig. 13.1) [25]. This algorithm guides decision-making by presenting possible muscular causes for scapular dysfunction and suggesting specific therapeutic strategies. Based on this algorithm, the scapulothoracic muscle dysfunction may be attributed to flexibility deficits in the soft tissue surrounding the scapula or altered scapular muscle performance [25]. Flexibility deficits or altered scapular muscle performance may be present after immobilization or at later stages of rehabilitation in patients with scapular fracture. Treatment for flexibility deficits may include manual soft tissue techniques and mobilization, manual stretching and mobilization with movement, and trigger point therapy. Strength training for muscle weakness or neuromuscular coordination training for neuromuscular deficits may effectively address altered scapular muscle performance [25]. Volitional muscle control of the scapular muscles, followed by co-contraction with selective activation of the weaker muscles (i.e., middle, lower trapezius or serratus anterior) with minimal activity of the hyperactive muscles (i.e., upper trapezius) may be initiated in the early phase of scapular muscle performance training. Therapeutic exercises can progress to general muscle strengthening exercises that may focus on activity or sport once scapular muscle balance is restored [25].

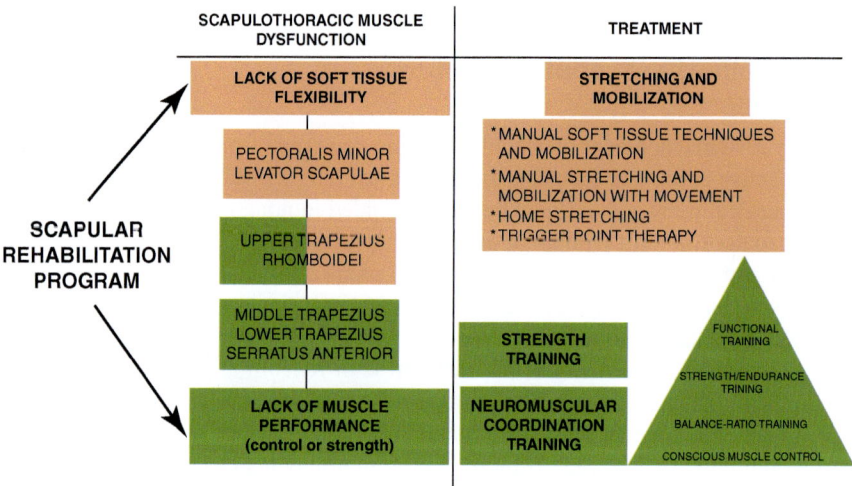

Fig. 13.1 Modified treatment algorithm for scapular dysfunction (originally from Ellenbecker and Cools [28]). In scapular rehabilitation, two pathways can be followed: orange pathway (management of lack of soft tissue flexibility, with presentation of most common muscles in which inflexibility occurs [left-orange], and accompanying treatment suggestions [right-orange] or green pathway (management of lack of muscle performance, with presentation of most common muscles in which control or strength problems occurs [left-green], and accompanying treatment suggestions [right-green]. (Reprinted from B. Castelein, B. Cagnie, A. Cools, Scapular muscle dysfunction associated with subacromial pain syndrome. J Hand Ther. 2017;30(2):136–46. with permission from Elsevier)

13.4 Rehabilitation After Surgical Fixation Following Scapular Fracture

The challenging nature of rehabilitation following surgical fixation for scapular fractures is owed to several factors, including the paucity of available research evidence, the multitude of fracture patterns and types, the mechanism involved and any concomitant injuries, the complexity of the scapular and shoulder anatomy involved, the interdependence between the cervical and thoracic spine and shoulder complex, the variety of surgical approaches utilized, and myriad surgeon preferences. Therefore, the physical therapist should base post-operative rehabilitation on tissue-healing principles, post-surgical precautions, ongoing surveillance for complications, patient response to treatment, and surgeon guidance.

Functional outcomes following surgical treatment of scapular fractures tend to be positive [26, 27]. In many ways, assuming patent fixation and appropriate stabilization, rehabilitation following surgery may proceed more aggressively and at a quicker pace than rehabilitation for conservative care, that is, nonsurgical treatment of scapular fractures. However, given the intimate location of the scapula and shoulder complex to the thorax, including visceral and neurovascular structures, relatively common occurrence of concomitant injuries, and potential complications of the surgery, the physical therapist should be vigilant in surveilling for possible post-operative complications, including infection, neurovascular compromise, nonunion, and evolving impairments outside of the scapula and shoulder complex.

The physical therapist may use the STAR-Shoulder rating system to assess the level of tissue irritability and match the goals and intensity of the intervention [7, 9] (Table 13.1) for the rehabilitation following surgical fixation. The sling may be limited to sleep and patient comfort, and the patient should be weaned entirely off by week 4 post-surgery to minimize the risk of shoulder and elbow stiffness. Rehabilitation following surgery should focus on early mobilization within pain tolerance to achieve full ROM, including passive and active assisted in the shoulder complex and active in the elbow, wrist, and hand, in all planes, and discontinuing any activity limitations by post-operative week 6 [5]. Assuming surgeon clearance, shoulder complex active range of motion in all planes and strength training with low resistance can begin as early as 4 weeks post-operatively. A more conservative approach to the rehabilitation process with an expanded and decelerated timeline is indicated when a more complicated surgery is performed, e.g., involving a deltoid or supraspinatus myotomy or release. Shoulder external rotation weakness is common after scapular fracture, especially with the Judet posterior approach, but also due to suprascapular nerve traction or compression caused by fracture displacement [5]. Activity modification and ROM restoration must precede any high-demand functional restoration [9]. The patient can safely progress to heavier resistance exercises with a focus on endurance and activity- and sport-specific training at weeks 8–12. When scapular dysfunction is present, the modified scapular dysfunction algorithm may be used to guide decision-making (Fig. 13.1) [25].

13.5 Conclusion

This chapter suggests rehabilitation strategies after scapular fracture, integrating available research evidence in shoulder and scapular dysfunction management with the primary pathoanatomical diagnosis. Physical therapists are best positioned to detect and treat musculoskeletal impairments associated with scapular fractures, including those managed conservatively and surgically.

References

1. Libby C, Frane N, Bentley TP. Scapula fracture. Treasure Island: StatPearls Publishing LLC; 2022.
2. Cole PA, Gauger EM, Schroder LK. Management of scapular fractures. J Am Acad Orthop Surg. 2012;20(3):130–41.
3. Reisch B, Fischer J. Rehabilitation of a patient with 'floating shoulder' and associated fractures: a case report. Physiother Theory Pract. 2012;28(7):542–51.
4. Sharma J, Maenza C, Myers A, Lehman EB, Karduna AR, Sainburg RL, et al. Clinical outcomes and shoulder kinematics for the "Gray zone" extra-articular scapula fracture in 5 patients. Int J Orthop. 2020;3(1):1017.
5. Limb D. Scapula fractures: a review. EFORT Open Rev. 2021;6(6):518–25.
6. Mahendraraj KA, Abboud J, Armstrong A, Austin L, Brolin T, Entezari V, et al. Predictors of acromial and scapular stress fracture after reverse shoulder arthroplasty: a study by the ases complications of rsa multicenter research group. J Shoulder Elb Surg. 2021;30(10):2296–305.
7. McClure PW, Michener LA. Staged approach for rehabilitation classification: shoulder disorders (star-shoulder). Phys Ther. 2015;95(5):791–800.
8. Schwank A, Blazey P, Asker M, Møller M, Hägglund M, Gard S, et al. 2022 Bern consensus statement on shoulder injury prevention, rehabilitation, and return to sport for athletes at all participation levels. J Orthop Sports Phys Ther. 2022;52(1):11–28.
9. Kareha SM, McClure PW, Fernandez-Fernandez A. Reliability and concurrent validity of shoulder tissue irritability classification. Phys Ther. 2021;101(3)
10. Kelley MJ, Shaffer MA, Kuhn JE, Michener LA, Seitz AL, Uhl TL, et al. Shoulder pain and mobility deficits: adhesive capsulitis. J Orthop Sports Phys Ther. 2013;43(5):A1–31.
11. Petersen EJ, Thurmond SM, Jensen GM. Severity, irritability, nature, stage, and stability (sinss): a clinical perspective. J Man Manip Ther. 2021;29(5):297–309.
12. Barakatt ET, Romano PS, Riddle DL, Beckett LA, Kravitz R. An exploration of maitland's concept of pain irritability in patients with low back pain. J Man Manip Ther. 2009;17(4):196–205.
13. Barakatt ET, Romano PS, Riddle DL, Beckett LA. The reliability of maitland's irritability judgments in patients with low back pain. J Man Manip Ther. 2009;17(3):135–40.
14. Somerville K, Walston Z, Marr T, Yake D. Treatment of shoulder pathologies based on irritability: a case series. Physiother Theory Pract. 2020;36(11):1266–74.
15. Mueller MJ, Maluf KS. Tissue adaptation to physical stress: a proposed "physical stress theory" to guide physical therapist practice, education, and research. Phys Ther. 2002;82(4):383–403.
16. Hart DL, Wang YC, Cook KF, Mioduski JE. A computerized adaptive test for patients with shoulder impairments produced responsive measures of function. Phys Ther. 2010;90(6):928–38.
17. Leggin BG, Michener LA, Shaffer MA, Brenneman SK, Iannotti JP, Williams GR Jr. The penn shoulder score: reliability and validity. J Orthop Sports Phys Ther. 2006;36(3):138–51.
18. Beaton D, Richards RR. Assessing the reliability and responsiveness of 5 shoulder questionnaires. J Shoulder Elb Surg. 1998;7(6):565–72.

19. Aldon-Villegas R, Ridao-Fernández C, Torres-Enamorado D, Chamorro-Moriana G. How to assess shoulder functionality: a systematic review of existing validated outcome measures. Diagnostics (Basel). 2021;11(5):845.
20. Kibler WB, Ludewig PM, McClure PW, Michener LA, Bak K, Sciascia AD. Clinical implications of scapular dyskinesis in shoulder injury: the 2013 consensus statement from the 'scapular summit'. Br J Sports Med. 2013;47(14):877–85.
21. Tate AR, McClure P, Kareha S, Irwin D, Barbe MF. A clinical method for identifying scapular dyskinesis, part 2: validity. J Athl Train. 2009;44(2):165–73.
22. McClure P, Tate AR, Kareha S, Irwin D, Zlupko E. A clinical method for identifying scapular dyskinesis, part 1: reliability. J Athl Train. 2009;44(2):160–4.
23. Seitz AL, McClure PW, Lynch SS, Ketchum JM, Michener LA. Effects of scapular dyskinesis and scapular assistance test on subacromial space during static arm elevation. J Shoulder Elb Surg. 2012;21(5):631–40.
24. Tate AR, McClure PW, Kareha S, Irwin D. Effect of the scapula reposition test on shoulder impingement symptoms and elevation strength in overhead athletes. J Orthop Sports Phys Ther. 2008;38(1):4–11.
25. Castelein B, Cagnie B, Cools A. Scapular muscle dysfunction associated with subacromial pain syndrome. J Hand Ther. 2017;30(2):136–46.
26. Schroder LK, Gauger EM, Gilbertson JA, Cole PA. Functional outcomes after operative management of extra-articular glenoid neck and scapular body fractures. J Bone Joint Surg Am. 2016;98(19):1623–30.
27. Tatro JM, Gilbertson JA, Schroder LK, Cole PA. Five to ten-year outcomes of operatively treated scapular fractures. J Bone Joint Surg Am. 2018;100(10):871–8.
28. Ellenbecker TS, Cools A. Rehabilitation of shoulder impingement syndrome and rotator cuff injuries: an evidence-based review. Br J Sports Med. 2010;44(5):319–27.

Index

A
Acromioclavicular injuries, 31
Acromion fractures, 17
   classification system, 82
   diagnosis, 81
   injury mechanism, 81, 82
   non-operative management, 82, 83
   operative management, 83–85
Adolescents
   complications, 31
   diagnosis, 28
   epidemiology, 27, 28
   treatment, 28–31
Anterior glenoid (AG) fractures, 62

B
Brachial plexus injuries, 31
Brodsky approach, 118, 123, 126

C
Children
   complications, 31
   diagnosis, 28
   epidemiology, 27, 28
   treatment, 28–31
Complex scapular fractures
   clinical setting, 111
   dominant limb
      clinical setting, 114, 117
      fixation strategy, 116, 118, 119
      preoperative planning, 114, 115, 118
      radiographic images and CT-Scan, 114, 115, 117
   humerus shaft
      clinical setting, 119
      fixation strategy, 121
      preoperative planning, 119, 120
      radiographic images and CT-scan, 119, 120
   non-dominant limb
      clinical setting, 111
      fixation strategy, 113, 114
      preoperative planning, 112
      3D CT-scan, 111, 112
   right multifragmentary fracture
      clinical setting, 121, 124
      fixation strategy, 123–126
      preoperative planning, 122–125
      radiographic images and CT scan, 121, 122, 124
Coracoid process fractures, 17
   anatomy, 73
   classification, 75
   injury mechanism, 74, 75
   prevalence, 73, 74
   treatment
      non-operative, 75
      operative, 76–81

D
Domestic violence, 27, 28

E
Entire glenoid (EG) fossa, 62–63

F
Fixation strategies
  caudal surface, 41
  cortical screws/cannulated screws, 41
  French bender, 41
  locking technology, 41
  pediatric Kocher clamps, 41
  reduction, 40
Floating flail chest, 22
  bilateral scapula fracture, 103, 106
  clavicle fixation, 105
  clavicle fracture and infraglenoid fracture, 102
  clinical presentation, 104
  glenopolar angle, 102
  incidence, 104
  mechanical ventilation, 104, 107
  non-operative treatment, 103–105
  open reduction and fracture fixation, 102, 103
  overview, 101
  postoperative care, 105
  prone positioning, 105
  rib fractures, 103
  scapula fixation, 105, 108
  surgical indications, 105
  treatment protocol, 104, 108
Floating shoulder, 22, 24
  complications, 98
  definition, 89, 90
  superior shoulder suspensory complex, 90–93
  surgical indications
    clavicular approach and fixation, 94, 95
    displacement, 93
    factors, 93
    operative stabilization, 93
    pain control and respiratory function, 93
    reduction instruments and implants, 96, 97
    rehabilitation program, 93
    scapular approach and fixation, 95, 96

G
Glenohumeral (GH) instability, *see* Glenoid fossa fractures; Glenoid rim fractures
Glenoid fossa fractures
  anatomy, 57, 58
  classification, 59–63
  injury mechanism, 58
  management
    anterior vertical axillary approach, 64–69
    deltopectoral approach, 64
    evaluation, 63
    prognosis, recovery, and satisfaction, 63
    rehabilitation protocol, 69
  physical examination, 59
  prevalence, 57
  radiographic workup, 59
Glenoid fractures, 28, 49
Glenoid rim fractures
  anatomy, 57, 58
  classification, 59–63
  injury mechanism, 58
  management
    anterior vertical axillary approach, 64–69
    deltopectoral approach, 64
    evaluation, 63
    prognosis, recovery, and satisfaction, 63
    rehabilitation protocol, 69
  physical examination, 59
  prevalence, 57
  radiographic workup, 59

I
Ideberg classification system, 60
Inferior glenoid (IG) fractures, 62

J
Judet approach
  deltoid sparing, 36, 37
  imaging, 33, 34
  infraspinatus sparing, 36, 37
  infraspinatus tenotomy, 37, 38
  posterior approach, 33–35
  posterior deltoid, 46
  prone positioning, 33
  reduction maneuvers and definitive fixation, 45
  triceps release, 37

N
Non-operative management
  outcomes, 24, 25
  patient selection, 21–23
  treatment protocol, 23, 24

Index

O

Open reduction and internal fixation (ORIF), 24, 28, 64

P

Patient-reported outcome measures (PROs), 138, 139
Periprosthetic scapular fracture
  epidemiology, 129–131
  risk factors, 129–131
  treatment, 132–134
Physical therapy, 138, 139
Pneumothorax, 31
Posterior glenoid (PG) fractures, 62

R

Rehabilitation
  conservative management, 139, 140
  physical therapy, 138, 139
  surgical fixation, 141
Reverse Judet approach, 38, 39
Reverse shoulder arthroplasty (RSA), 18
  epidemiology, 129–131
  risk factors, 129–131
  treatment, 132–134
Rib fractures, 31

S

Scapular assistance test, 139
Scapular dyskinesis test, 139
Scapular fractures
  Ada and Miller classification, 13
  anatomy of, 2–5
  AO/OTA classification, 10, 11
  Bartoníček classification, 14, 17
  biomechanics, injury mechanism, and epidemiology, 6–8
  in children and adolescents
    complications, 31
    diagnosis, 28
    epidemiology, 27, 28
    treatment, 28–31
  classification system
    extra-articular fractures, 9
    intra-articular fractures, 9
  deltopectoral, 39, 40
  development of, 1, 2
  Euler and Rüedi classification, 10, 12
  Eyres classification, 16, 17
  fixation strategies (*see* Fixation strategies)
  Goss classification, 13, 14
  Hardegger classification, 14
  Harley classification, 10, 11, 13
  Ideberg classification, 14, 15
  Judet approach (*see* Judet approach)
  Kuhn classification, 17
  lateral window and minimally invasive, 38
  Levy classification, 18
  minimally invasive approaches, 42
  Naniwa classification, 17
  neck and body
    fixation strategies, 48, 49
    operative approach, 45–48
    patient history, 50–54
  non-operative management
    outcomes, 24, 25
    patient selection, 21–23
    treatment protocol, 23, 24
  Ogawa classification, 16, 17
  Petit classification, 10
  rehabilitation (*see* Rehabilitation)
  Reverse Judet approach, 38, 39
Scapular reposition test, 139
Sports activities, 27
Staged Algorithm for Rehabilitation Classification (STAR-Shoulder), 138
Superior glenoid (SG) fossa fractures, 61

V

Van Noort approach, 121

GPSR Compliance

The European Union's (EU) General Product Safety Regulation (GPSR) is a set of rules that requires consumer products to be safe and our obligations to ensure this.

If you have any concerns about our products, you can contact us on ProductSafety@springernature.com

In case Publisher is established outside the EU, the EU authorized representative is:

Springer Nature Customer Service Center GmbH
Europaplatz 3
69115 Heidelberg, Germany

Batch number: 08667368

Printed by Printforce, the Netherlands